THE COMPLETE GUIDE TO

YOGA FOR FITNESS PROFESSIONALS

Debbie Lawrence & Conrad Paul

BLOOMSBURY
LONDON · NEW DELHI · NEW YORK · SYDNEY

Note
While every effort has been made to ensure that the content of this book is as technically accurate and as sound as possible, neither the author nor the publishers can accept responsibility for any injury or loss sustained as a result of the use of this material.

Published by Bloomsbury Publishing Plc
50 Bedford Square
London WC1B 3DP
www.bloomsbury.com
Bloomsbury is a trademark of Bloomsbury Publishing Plc

First edition 2014
Copyright © 2014 Debbie Lawrence and Conrad Paul
ISBN (print): 978-1-4081-8721-0
ISBN (epub): 978-1-4729-0967-1
ISBN (epdf): 978-1-4729-1147-6

All rights reserved. No part of this publication may be reproduced in any form or by any means – graphic, electronic or mechanical, including photocopying, recording, taping or information storage and retrieval systems – without the prior permission in writing of the publishers.

Debbie Lawrence and Conrad Paul have asserted their rights under the Copyright, Design and Patents Act, 1988, to be identified as the authors of this work.

A CIP catalogue record for this book is available from the British Library.

Acknowledgements
Cover photograph © Getty Images
Inside photographs © Grant Pritchard with the exception of
the following; pp. 6, 35, 78, 90, 132 and 192 © Shutterstock
Illustrations by Mark Silver

Commissioning Editor: Charlotte Croft
Editor: Sarah Cole
Design: James Watson
Typesetting and page layouts: Susan McIntyre

This book is produced using paper that is made from wood grown in managed, sustainable forests. It is natural, renewable and recyclable. The logging and manufacturing processes conform to the environmental regulations of the country of origin.

Typeset in 10.75 on 14pt Adobe Caslon

Printed and bound in China by C&C Offset Printing Co

10 9 8 7 6 5 4 3 2 1

CONTENTS

Acknowledgements		4
PART ONE	YOGA HISTORY, PHILOSOPHY AND HATHA YOGA PRACTICE	7
Chapter 1	Introduction to yoga history	9
Chapter 2	The body and mind according to yoga	27
Chapter 3	Hatha yoga	53
Chapter 4	Practising asana – the first part of Hatha yoga	57
Chapter 5	Pranayama – breath work/regulation and control	148
Chapter 6	Mudras, bandhas and kriyas	162
Chapter 7	Session structure and general hatha flow sequence	172
PART TWO	APPLYING YOGA TO MODERN LIVING, AND THE SEQUENCES	193
Chapter 8	Yoga, fitness and health	194
Chapter 9	Yoga philosophy in modern living	211
Chapter 10	Yoga sequences by Conrad Paul	219
References		227
Glossary of terms		229
Appendices		232
1 Passive relaxation script 1		232
2 Active relaxation script		232
3 Passive relaxation script 2		234
4 Healing relaxation script		235
5 Simple chakra meditation script		236
Index		237

ACKNOWLEDGEMENTS

I have co-written this book as both a fitness professional and an integrative counsellor. I am a student of life who has an interest in the many different and alternative philosophies and approaches to healthy living and ageing.

I am not a yoga guru. I am continually learning and growing. I have a passion for sharing what I learn and what I know. I am truly thankful that my career and my life offer many opportunities for me to write, teach, learn and share.

My hope is the book captures the 'essence' of yoga; which to me, as a therapist and human being, equates to being the best one can be and a decent person.

Special thanks to:

- my partner Joe for his ongoing love, support and uplifting spirit
- my mum, dad, brother and sisters for their contribution to my life
- my therapy teachers and mentors – Sheila Norris, Graz Amber, Mike Berry, Marilia Angove
- my heroes of the therapy world: Carl Rogers, Carl Jung, Fritz Perls, Irvine Yalom, Eric Berne, Sigmund Freud (to name but a few)
- my yoga teachers and colleagues: Sue Moore, Annie Vincent, Conrad Paul, Alex Carr, Pippa Yarwoth-Cleeton
- my co-author Conrad, who has a far greater knowledge of yoga traditions and practice, and without whom I would not have been able to write this book
- the team at Bloomsbury who are always supportive and work to make ideas and projects happen
- everyone involved in the photoshoot for their time and energy to help the day run smoothly. Debra Stuart of Premier Global and the team at Premier Training International Finsbury Park for providing the venue; and models, Alex Carr, Emese Pomesanksi, Annie Vincent; photographer, Grant Pritchard and Sarah Cole from Bloomsbury.

Thank you, thank you, thank you!
Wishing you all good things,

Debbie Lawrence MA BA (Hons)
PG Dip Integrative counselling

ACKNOWLEDGEMENTS

I have written this book from the perspective of a modern-day yoga practitioner. After founding my yoga teacher training school 'Yoga Professionals' in 2007, my own practices, growth and teaching have developed through all the reflections I have received from every student that has trained with me, and has gone on to shine the light of yoga. I have a deep passion and love of yoga and I hope that through this book I will pass on to you the reality of 'modern-day practices', stemming from the ancient wisdoms of the yogis that went before.

I am not a guru, but I believe the guru is within each and every one of us, and I hope through this book those who read it will awaken their own curiosity and self-realisation that life can be joyous, even when there are moments of darkness.

Special thanks to:

- my mum who has always been the ultimate inspiration in my life as she filled me with so much love
- my best friend Yod (Pacharapong Suntanaphan), a beautiful soul
- my brother Wayne, a great yoga teacher himself, who pushed me towards the light of yoga, and Jason, who is a kind soul who does not understand how much yoga he has in him, without even studying the practice
- my friends, Hala Thurston, Debbie Hudson, Clodagh O'Reilly, Tina Iannou and Lesley Ann Oakes, for always being there for me no matter what
- my co-lecturers at Yoga Professionals: Renu Singh, Sujatha Menon, and especially Annie Vincent for all her support and love
- my teachers in education, Mrs Parkes and Dr Catherine Kerr, both of whom have no idea how inspirational they have been in my personal growth
- my co-author Debbie, without whom this book would never have happened
- the yoga teachers and fellow yogis who I have studied, met, and trained with
- all the swamis and gurus, with my deepest love for Swami Sadasivananda for his shining light and love, Om Swamiji, you will always be my guru
- George Harrison and Crispian Mills for their musical influences that have engaged my journey into Bhakti Yoga, Hari Krishna!
- the hugging mother 'Amma' for her incredible life force and energy

108 salutations and thanks to you all for your special qualities that have given me so much joy and love in life.

Om Namah Shivaya!

Conrad Paul – Yoga Acharia

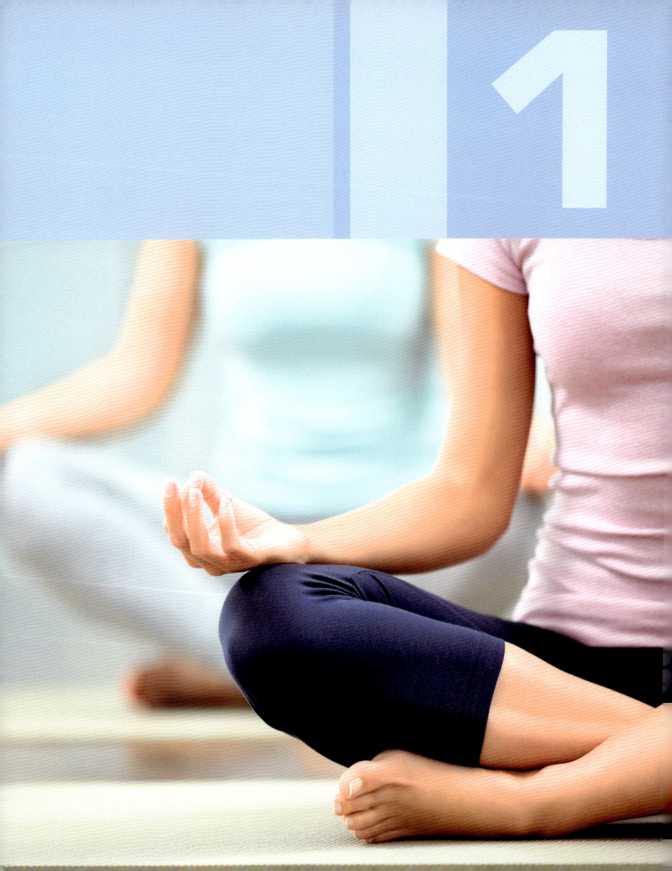

PART ONE

YOGA HISTORY, PHILOSOPHY AND HATHA YOGA PRACTICE

If you were to ask the everyday person in the Western hemisphere the question 'what is yoga?' the most probable answer would be that it is a series of physical postures, or a form of exercise system that originated from India. This notion of 'yoga' is the practice of Hatha yoga – one pathway.

Yoga is actually a spiritual discipline and features in traditions of Hinduism, Jainism and certain schools of Buddhism; even if they do not necessarily use the word. It is a scientific, artistic, philosophical and physical system where the shared goal is to achieve Samadhi (ecstasy) and union with the Divine through a variety of practices. Emphasis may be placed upon such things as devotion to a higher power, meditation to still the mind and many other practices that may lead to liberation (moksha/kaivalya) from the cycle of birth, death and suffering, and attain oneness with the Universe, (Satyananda, 1980).

Far from being just an exercise system, yoga helps us connect to our true selves and true nature. Embracing both inner and outer realities helps bring definite results to those who practise. Continuous and dedicated daily practices of the various aspects of yoga, including moral conduct, attitude to others, withdrawal of the senses from the surrounding world, can help to bring a transformation that goes beyond exercise. The only way to understand yoga is through practice and experience, (Sivananda, 1986).

Traditionally, yoga is a method of joining the individual self with the Divine, Cosmic Consciousness or Universal Spirit (some would use the word God). The aspirant or practitioner (one who aspires to advancement) known in ancient times as the sadhaka, who, depressed at seeing and experiencing the same mundane existence, birth after birth, turns their attention towards the Supreme Soul or Paramatma, (Satyananda, 1969).

To put this in context, the average person's mind is often cluttered with the trivialities of consumer materialism, celebrity gossip, media brainwashing and chit-chat, so much so that one's true nature is not realised.

Sat Chit Ananda (translated from Sanskrit) means Truth, Consciousness, Bliss. According to yoga, our true consciousness or nature is the Truth (higher power) which is Blissful. Over the history of humanity's evolution we have advanced, some might say, in technology and industry, but this inner Truth has for many been forgotten. Instead, people spend endless years (and possibly lifetimes) ignoring their inner True Self (Satchitananda).

The ancient accomplished yogis, known as rishis (seers), would sit for hours in meditation day after day, and were so adept at calming the constant idle chit-chat of the mind that they were able to see things inwardly through the power of meditation. These great seers were able to observe things that others could not. In deep meditation they (so the yoga traditions believe) could see the worlds and planes of existence beyond this one, which gave them proof that our lives are based around pleasure and pain, which through the action of karma creates a never-ending cycle of birth and death. This loop keeps each individual's atman (soul) trapped in a constant cycle of misery and pain, life after life. The rishis saw that the life of each person who forgot their True Self would be based around fulfillment of the ahamkara (ego), and so yoga was passed down to teach humanity the true 'meaning of life' and to give each one of us the opportunity to learn the true purpose of incarnation, which is a life of bliss and happiness, (Feuerstein, 1998).

INTRODUCTION TO YOGA HISTORY

Today, many might say the world is in chaos. More and more people are turning to yoga to stop the constant stresses and related consequences on modern day mankind and planet earth. If we believe yoga's teachings (that everything is meant to be); then the lineage of yoga teachers has to expand at a 21st century rate to raise consciousness and help save the world from the possible darkness looming. The more people practise yoga, the more vibrant and loving the world will be. Trust that the lineage of yoga has evolved and so have the teachings. Yoga is as relevant today as when it was first born through the eyes of the Rishi's (seers). It is a gift to mankind.

By Conrad Paul and with reference to the teachings of Satyananda, 1980

WHAT IS YOGA?

Yoga stems from Hindu spirituality and is one of the six philosophical schools of thought or Darshana. An exact definition is difficult to articulate but the word 'yoga' stems from the Sanskrit root word, '*yuj*' which translated means '*yoke*' or '*to join*'.

Other definitions of the word 'yoga' include:
- To come together
- To unite
- To attain that which was previously unattainable
- To be one with the divine
- To be present in every action and every moment

Within yoga, the idea of that which must be joined is one's 'attention', which normally flits from object to object, (Feurstein, 1998). This is the mind, which is blocked by obstacles known as kleshas, including avidya (ignorance), which prevent us from knowing the truth of self, the divine within. To remove avidya, we need to surrender to a higher consciousness or higher being, the all-knowing source, the higher 'seer' Isvara. Isvara is represented by the symbol or mantra 'Om'; chanting the mantra Om is one path to connecting and building a relationship with Isvara, (Desikachar 1999:129). (Mind, kleshas, avidya, mantras and Om are discussed in chapter 2).

THE PATHS OF YOGA

The path to yoga, or the defined joining and union of mind, body and spirit can occur in different ways. There are different paths, for different people. The ancient seers understood that the differing natures of individuals needed alternative options to achieving liberation and thus different paths to yoga evolved. *The Bhagavad Gita* cites four paths (Jnana, Bhakti, Karma and Raja). Desikachar, (1999) describes additional paths (Mantra, Kriya, Hatha, Tantra and Kundalini), which represent the evolution of yoga practice from its earlier origins to modern-day practice. (The history of yoga is discussed on page 13).

For some, selfless service will form the path (Karma); for others reading and introspection (Jnana path); others may join through devotion to a deity and/or chanting and singing (Bhakti and Mantra paths); while some will join through meditative connection with the divine (Raja path) and others will connect through more physical practices – asana (Hatha).

Regardless of the path descriptions and activities, they will all, according to yoga philosophy, eventually lead to other paths and to Raja yoga – the royal road and king of all practices. The teachings which inform the practice of each path may be different, but ultimately they all lead to the same thing – union and joining of the seen, physical matter (Prakriti) with the seer, the perceiver, source of consciousness (Purusa) with the divine within (Isvara).

KARMA YOGA

Karma means 'action' and this is the path of selfless service to others; the giving of your time and skills to help others without wanting or expecting reward. For example, during a stay at an ashram (yoga monastery) guests are required to dedicate a small amount of their time to the upkeep and running of the ashram, this is also known as Seva, or service, (Sivananda, 1986). A Karma yogi attempts to see the divine in all things.

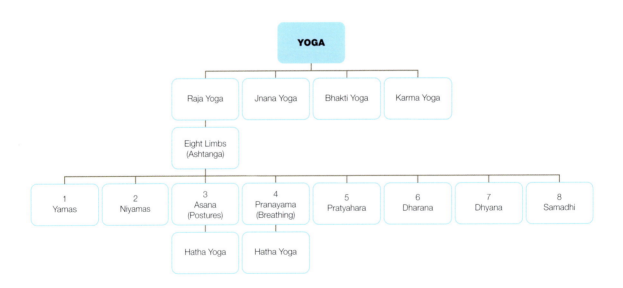

Figure 1.1 This represents a hierarchy of the origins of yoga, the four paths, the eight limbs and the evolution of 'Hatha yoga' from these historical origins.

Karma yoga is a central theme within *The Bhagavad Gita* (see page 24) and also within the yoga sutras (see page 18), which offers the following definition:

'We must involve ourselves through action, but leave the rest to God and expect nothing'.
(Desikachar, 1999:137)

BHAKTI YOGA

Bhakti yoga is the yoga of devotion and service to a divine being. Chanting, singing, regular prayers, japa (repeating a mantra or name of God) and celebrations are all forms of Bhakti yoga. Jaya Ganesha is a twice-daily chant of the Sivananda devotees, which calls upon Lord Ganesha, the remover of obstacles, and many other deities to help them clear the way to Samadhi or spiritual bliss. The maha (great) mantra of the Hari Krishna movement is chanted to help liberate the aspirant by the repetition of 'Hari Rama, Hari Rama, Rama Rama, Hari Hari, Hari Krishna, Hari Krishna, Krishna Krishna, Hari Hari', which is used to draw the mental focus towards Lord Krishna, an avatar (incarnation) of Lord Vishnu, considered the sustainer of the universe in Hindu mythology. The japa (repetition) of the mantra helps to focus the mind into a state known as 'eka grata' (one pointed), in the direction of the deity Krishna also known as Hari, this continued focus helps to still the chatter of the mind which is considered in yoga to be one of the reasons we cannot find peace and tranquility, and thus cannot rest in our own true nature, (Satyananda, 1969).

MANTRA YOGA

A mantra can be a single syllable, a number of syllables or a verse, that is chanted regularly to offer protection to the person to whom it was given. The mantra is usually given by a guru to a student when they know exactly what the student needs. Mantra yoga is believed to have the same effects as Bhakti and Jnana yoga, (Desikachar, 1999:136).

JNANA YOGA

Jnana in Sanskrit means knowledge, and is the path of wisdom and intellect. Through the study of ancient texts, philosophical discussion, intellectual debate with others and introspection, 'that which lies within us' is revealed. This is the path of Jnana yoga, (Desikachar, 1999:135).

Sivananda (1986) suggests this to be the most direct of the paths, but also the most difficult as the aspirant needs to be firmly grounded in the other disciplines before attempting it. This form of yoga is for the more studious personality.

RAJA YOGA

Raja yoga, also known as the 'royal path', is the journey towards personal enlightenment. The mind is systematically analysed and techniques are applied to bring it under control (reduce its restlessness) and achieve Samadhi or a higher state of consciousness (the king within).

Raja yoga is about recognising the divine, the 'king' within ourselves and allowing him to take his rightful place. This 'king' may be known as God, Isvara or Purusha or as the same divine being celebrated in Bhakti yoga, (Desikachar, 1999:136).

KRIYA YOGA

The yoga sutras describe Kriya yoga as a whole spectrum of practices. The Kriya yoga system of yoga was revived in modern times by Lahiri Mahasaya, (*c.* 1861). It was Paramahansa Yogananda who brought it into widespread public awareness.

The system consists of a number of yogic techniques that hasten the practitioner's spiritual development and help to bring about a profound state of tranquility and God-communion, (Yogananda, 2006). Kriya yoga consists of:

- **Tapas**: discipline. Includes practices such as asana and pranayama to remove blocks and physical obstacles.
- **Svadhyaya**: self-study. Asking ourselves questions to explore who we are and what is our purpose.
- **Ishvara Pranidhana**: surrender. Surrendering to the divine and dedication to a higher principle or purpose, '*action (is) not motivated by outcome*', (Desikachar, 1999:137).

These three combined practices are the Kriya path and lead to a reduction in the kleshas (spiritual obstacles, which include avidya) and bring about a feeling of meditative absorption, (Yogananda, 2006).

HATHA, KUNDALINI AND TANTRA YOGA

In Hatha, Kundalini and Tantra yoga practice, Kundalini is a central concept, as are the nadis chakras, sushumna and prana.

- **Kundalini yoga** emphasises the concept of Kundalini.
- **Hatha yoga** emphasises the joining of Ha and tha (sun and moon, and masculine and feminine energies). Hatha is believed to be a pathway to Raja yoga.
- **Tantra yoga** emphasises the containment and direction of certain energies to remove obstacles, rather than wasting these energies.

Desikachar describes Kundalini (see chapter 2) as an obstacle or another form of avidya (see chapter 2) and suggests there is much confusion regarding the concept of Kundalini. To fully understand Kundalini, it is suggested that one needs a wealth of practical experience, sound knowledge and also a clear understanding of the Sanskrit language; all of which 'are often lacking', (Desikachar, 1999:139).

The teachings which inform the practice of each path are different, but ultimately, they are all aiming towards the same goal: the union of the body and the inner divinity.

THE SIX SCHOOLS OF INDIAN PHILOSOPHY – THE SHAD DARSHANAS

Yoga is one of the six fundamental systems of Indian thought or darshana, which translated means 'to see' or 'a way of seeing', and has its origins in the ancient texts called the Vedas, (Desikachar, 1999:5).

The six darshanas are:
1. **Yoga**
2. **Samkhya**
3. **Nyaya**
4. **Vaisesika**
5. **Vedanta**
6. **Mimamsa**

The six schools of Indian philosophy are the ancient teachings regarding various aspects of the Universe ranging from subjects such as: quantum physics, mathematics and the science of life, known as Ayurveda.

1. **Yoga**: Allied with Samkhya, the school focuses on the studies of all aspects of human personality. It teaches one how to control the modifications of the mind through practice of meditation, and detachment through surrender to a higher consciousness. Founded by Patanjali, it follows the Samkhya philosophy but adds the belief of God.

2. **Samkhya**: A dualistic philosophy that believes in the co-existent and interdependent realities – the conscious Purusa and the unconscious Prakriti. Samkhya philosophy explains the dynamics of the body and nature of mind. It is the mother of mathematics as well as Ayurveda (the Indian system for health and healing) and is indeed the very basis of Eastern philosophy. Founded by Kapila it is based on the 25 elements of creation.

3. **Nyaya**: The school of logic that was set up by the sage Guatama. It deals with philosophical reasoning and debate.

4. **Vaisesika**: This school discusses seven major topics: substance, quality, action, generality, uniqueness, inherence and non-existence. This school established the theory of atomic structure. Founded by Kananda it is a supplementary to Nyaya and focuses on time, space, cause and matter.

5. **Vedanta**: This school teaches that self-realisation is the actual goal of life, the essence of the self is the ever-existent consciousness and bliss. The self is free from all limitations and is essentially Brahman, the Supreme Consciousness. Non-duality (Advaita Vedanta) by Adi Shankara is one of the most popular forms of Vedanta and subjects such as maya or the veil of illusion/deceit are within its teachings. Founded by Badarayana it emphasises knowledge from the Vedas.

6. **Mimamsa**: Offers guidelines for practical application of Vedantic theory. This school is foremost in the analysis of sound and mantra, (Feuerstein, 2003). Founded by Jaimini it focuses on the Vedic religious rituals, (Chanchani and Chanchani, 1995).

THE HISTORY OF YOGA

The history of yoga spans many millennia. The roots of yoga can be traced back roughly 5,000 years, to the Brahmin priests of ancient India. Originally, yoga was passed on as an oral tradition through an unbroken lineage of gurus and disciples working closely together to preserve the early sacred teachings (Vedas and Upanishads). Over the centuries, it has evolved and taken many different forms.

Through experimentation, the symbolism of the early texts have been expanded and developed by yoga practitioners and handed down through the generations, (Feuerstein, 2003).

Yoga is not a religion or a renunciation of religion. Yoga does not demand anything of the individual other than to live a meaningful life of goodness and equanimity that furthers one's own development without harming others. Transcending mere physical exercise, yoga incorporates relaxation, breathing and energy components, along with awareness of the self, physically, mentally and spirituality, (Satyananda, 1969).

THE FOUR SECTS, DHARMA AND RIGHTEOUSNESS

In ancient India, and until the eventual outlawing by Gandhi, India had four sects or 'castes' of people. This caste system gave order to the peoples of India and through this order their civilisation grew and thrived. The four sects or castes were:
1. the priests, known as Brahmins (the highest order)
2. the warrior caste
3. the farmers
4. the workers.

The caste you were born into determined your place in the hierarchy. Dharma in Sanskrit means righteousness, or duty, and within this caste system, people knew their place and duty in society and lived according to their 'destined' caste, (Feuerstein, 1998). The priests were considered the highest of the castes as they were considered the closest to the Divine, the warriors were born with the duty of protecting and serving, the farmers with the duty of producing the food, and the workers performing duties to serve the other castes.

This system, which was maintained for millennia, meant that one's status at birth dictated one's place and duty in society. In many countries (including the UK) people are born into families of a certain status and, as such, have privileges afforded to them by birth rather than accomplishment.

A brief overview of the main texts and historical periods follows.

THE VEDAS AND THE VEDIC PERIOD
Estimated historical date: 4500–2500 BCE

Veda is the Sanskrit term, meaning 'knowledge'. The Veda (book of knowledge) is the holy book of Hinduism. The Veda was based around the Brahmin priest's connection to different deities through external ritual, sacrifice, astrology and the plant/drug Soma.

There are four books that form the Veda (commonly known as the Vedas), these are:
1. Rig Veda
2. Yajur Veda
3. Sama Veda
4. Atharva Veda.

The texts consist of hymns that were originally passed to the ancient rishis (seers) from Hiranyagarbha (the golden womb of knowledge of the universe). This information is considered to be from the Supreme Consciousness or Paramatman (parama: 'highest'; atma: 'soul'), which is considered to have been 'revealed' (shruti), and then passed on to the Brahmin priests.

The earliest book is the Rig Veda, a collection of 1,017 hymns dedicated to a wide assortment of gods. In Hindu mythology, the Veda has existed from before the beginning of time. It was carefully preserved by Brahma (the four-faced god of creation), during the dissolution of the last universe, and then given to humanity once again when the world was recreated. Traditionally these sacred teachings were then taught in the form of oral hymns to 'Brahmin priests in training', thus maintaining the Indian caste system of the time, (Feuerstein, 1998).

> *I will tell you the brave deeds of Indra, Lord of thunder!*
> *He killed the dragon, He made the waters flow*
> *He broke open the mountain*
> *Indra is the Lord of all things living and inanimate.*
>
> (Griffith, 1891)

THE UPANISHADS AND THE PRE-CLASSICAL OR POST-VEDIC PERIOD
Estimated historical date: 1500–1000 BCE

The Upanishads came about as a reform or 'culmination of the Vedas' to allow ordinary people to be introduced to the internalised ritualism or 'inner sacrifice' (antar yajna) without the need for a priest. The authors of the texts are unknown, and the number of the writings vary, as some Upanishads were written at later dates in history. The texts were considered to be ways to the Vedas. In the Upanishads, more emphasis was placed on personal worship, devotion, and the replacement of sacrifice with worship.

The term Upanishad is derived from upa (near), ni (down) and s(h)ad (to sit), i.e., sitting down near. Groups of pupils would sit near the teacher to learn from him and the secret doctrine. In the quietude of the forest hermitages the Upanishad thinkers pondered on the problems of deepest concerns and communicated their knowledge to suit pupils near them, (Feuerstein, 1998).

The four main concepts of the Upanishad teachings were that:

1. We are our own universe and are the same as the ultimate Universe
2. Without acknowledgement of the Atman or soul we cannot liberate from the cycle of birth and death
3. Our destiny is determined by our thoughts and actions, and
4. Without liberation one will reincarnate again and again, due to karma, (Feuerstein, 1998).

The Upanishads taught inner practices (such as meditation) over sacrificial offerings; which helped form the foundations of Hinduism as it is known today.

> *He who knows Brahaman while on earth has achieved his sole object of life; they who do not, suffer great misfortune. The wise perceiving the oneness of all beings in Atman, rise above sensory phenomena and are immortal.*
>
> Kenopanishad Upanishad 2:5, (Satyananda, 1975)

This Divine being, the creator and the all-pervading soul of this universe, resides in the heart of all living beings. Those who meditate on Him with heart, mind and intellect attain immortality.

Shevtashvatara Upanishad 4:17, (Satyananda, 1975)

The bright space, familiar to all, is in the heart. Within that the intelligent Immortal and radiant soul (Purusha) exists who is realised and worshipped through meditation and knowledge.

Taittiriya Upanishad 6:1, (Satyananda, 1975)

THE CLASSICAL PERIOD – THE YOGA SUTRAS OF PATANJALI
Estimated historical date: 1000 BCE –100 BCE

The classical period was a time when the six schools of yoga philosophy were competing for intellectual supremacy, (Feuerstein, 1998). During this period the 'Yoga Sutras of Patanjali' were written. The focus of the sutras (discussed later in this chapter) were on meditation and stillness of the mind, alongside ethical guidelines and mystical powers, which are the more famous aspects of the teachings, all aimed at liberation or moksha from the cycle of life and death caused by karma which has occurred through deeds from previous incarnations, (Feuerstein, 2003).

THE POST-CLASSICAL PERIOD – TANTRA
Estimated historical date: is 1500–1000 BCE

The Tantric period placed a focus on the feminine psychic cosmic energy (Shakti) and, drawing upon previous texts from the Vedas of goddess worship, (Feuerstein, 1998), they began to evolve the use of the 'body as a temple', from which Hatha yoga practices later evolved.

There are two factions of Tantra called left-handed and right-handed Tantrics. Tantra became unpopular due to the left-handed Tantric acts of the five Ms:

1. **Madya** (wine)
2. **Mamsa** (meat)
3. **Matsya** (fish)
4. **Mudra** (parched grain)
5. **Maithuna** (coition).

These five acts went against most other yoga traditions, as the left-handed Tantrics would practise the five Ms as a form of yoga.

The right-handed Tantric practices of symbolism, rather than taking the five Ms literally, are what helped shape the modern-day Hatha yoga. The Tantric masters aspired to create a body that they called 'adamantine' – a body not made of flesh but of the immortal substance: the Light.

Instead of viewing the body as a tube doomed for decay and death, the Tantrics viewed it as a dwelling place for God or the Divine. Viewed as a 'whole body event', Tantra brought the idea of the 'body as a temple' into yoga, (Feuerstein, 1998).

MODERN DAY YOGA – HATHA YOGA
Estimated historical date: 1700 CE–present day

After the British Empire invaded India many of its treasures were revealed to the West, including its philosophies, ideals, beliefs and religions, (Singleton, 2010). Beyond the classical yoga schools that taught meditation and self-study, a popular form of yoga with 'effort' arose – Hatha yoga.

'Yoga is India's greatest gift to the West'.
Krishnamacharya, in Forstater and Manuel (2002:15)

As people began to travel more, Hatha yoga grew, and the export of books and ideas also allowed the teachings to expand into the world. Due to the difficulty in sitting in meditation for long periods, and the energetic nature of the Western world, effort-based Hatha yoga became the more common view of what yoga is today over the more classical Raja yoga of meditation, (Singleton, 2010).

Hatha yoga is a very small part of the full spectrum of yoga and is mostly a pathway to older more established systems. Hatha yoga practices and traditions are explored and discussed later in this section.

Yoga is a huge part of a spiritual heritage that has been evolving in the West since the flower-power days of the 1960s. After spending time in India visiting the spiritual guru Maharishi Mahesh Yogi, the Beatles' music took on 'Peace and Love' elements, and brought the teachings and practices of yoga into the mainstream, (Kozin, 2007).

But even before then, from the early part of the last century, some great yogis came to the West during times of darkness in the so-called Western 'civilisation', and introduced the philosophies that promoted peace, not war, as well as some of the different forms of yoga.

Swami Vishnu Devananda a direct disciple of Swami Sivananda, flew his tiny aeroplane of peace over the Berlin wall scattering flowers in East Berlin in the hope of promoting union over division. Swami Satchidananda wowed the hippy children of Woodstock with his chants of 'Om', and George Harrison introduced the world to Sri Prabhupada and the Hari Krishna movement, which had worldwide number one records with the Hari Krishna Mantra, the album *Goddess of Fortune* and George Harrison's 'My Sweet Lord', which incorporated the chant of Hari Krishna within its lyrics, exposing millions worldwide to the Eastern philosophy of Bhakti yoga (the yoga of chanting and devotion). Since then Yoga in the West has gone from strength to strength in its different incarnations from Transcendental Meditation, Bhakti, Hatha, and Kundalini to name just a few.

Yoga practices have proven to give direct and real benefits to people from all walks of life regardless of their spiritual aspirations. The power and effectiveness of Yoga comes from its holistic approach and its various styles, or types, to which end the different personality traits of each individual can find the one Yoga to suit them in bringing harmony and unification within. Yoga has been used as part of the treatment for diseases such as: asthma, arthritis, diabetes, digestive disorders, blood pressure problems and other chronic health conditions. It has also been used by some as an alternative to drugs offered by conventional medicine. Its contribution to improving mental health and its use in overcoming common addictions such as drugs, alcohol and tobacco has also been researched and published.

YOGA THERAPY

Yoga therapy has been proven by medical scientists to directly influence the systems and organs of the body by balancing the nervous and endocrine systems. Research is continuing and its efficacy is continually being confirmed, (Desikachar 1995).
- Asanas (yoga postures) can help remove the physical discomforts accumulated from everyday life.
- Relaxation gives us essential time off and allows moments of clarity to be revealed.

To respect all forms of yoga is to be the true yogi (a human being who is committed to the practice of yoga). To give thanks to all the yogis who came before us is honoring the true lineage of yoga, for yoga is not a style or a statement; it is a personal practice of love and compassion. Take from yoga whatever suits you as a human being and here begin your journey.

For those ignorant of Raja Yoga, wandering in the darkness of too many options, compassionate Svatmarama gives the light of Hatha.

Hatha Yoga Pradipika, Svatmarama,
Ch 1 vs. 3, (Akers, 2002).

THE YOGA SUTRAS OF PATANJALI

The yoga sutras, attributed to Maharishi (great seer) Patanjali, are a set of 196 aphorisms or threads, short phrases designed to be easy to memorise. In times gone by and even today, students of Raja yoga would memorise the sutras to use as a daily practice through exploration of the prescription to liberation. Though brief, the yoga sutras are an enormously influential work just as relevant for yoga philosophy and practice today, as it was when it was written, (Satyananda, 1976).

The yoga sutras are of an uncertain date, probably between 200 BCE and 200 CE. Little historic information is available on Patanjali, also known as the 'father of yoga', beyond legend and myth. His translation of the ancient scriptures is considered to have brought yoga to the masses.

Patanjali defines yoga as the settling of the mind back into an undisturbed state, where the self can be realised. This is unlike the normal mental condition where the mind identifies with what disturbs it, (Feuerstein, 2003). See chapter 2 for more discussion of the mind.

The sutras are set out in four chapters:
1. **Samadhi Pada** (contemplation: consciousness and super consciousness). Deals with the state of samadhi (ecstasy).
2. **Sadhana Pada** (practice: ways to attain yoga). Deals with how samadhi may be achieved, which includes the famous eight limbs of yoga (discussed on page 10 of this chapter).
3. **Vibhuti Pada** (properties and powers). Deals with the definition of the three meditative limbs of yoga (Dharana, Dhyana and Samadhi), the fruits of practice and the supernatural powers that may arise.

4. **Kaivalya Pada** (liberation, emancipation and freedom) – deals with the goal of yoga, Kaivalya, or the ability to discriminate between things of matter and the Divine.

B.K.S. Iyengar, one of the most well known and influential teachers of yoga in the West describes the four padas as corresponding to the four stages of life or asramas, the three qualities of nature, gunas (sattva, tapas and rajas – see page 26) and the four aims of living or life, purusarthas (1996:3).

THE EIGHT LIMBS OF YOGA (ALSO KNOWN AS ASHTANGA YOGA)

The Sanskrit word '*Ashta*' means eight and '*Anga*' means limbs.

> This is not to be confused with Ashtanga Vinyasa Karma, a Hatha yoga practice, rather than Raja yoga more commonly practised.

Patanjali's eight limbs of yoga form the ethical conduct and moral guidance for the yogi to adhere to for the achievement of the goal of Bliss/Absolute Superconscious state/Samadhi, written in Sanskrit as Satchitananda. They are found in the text of the yoga sutras of Patanjali.

The first four limbs concentrate on refining our personalities and behaviour, gaining mastery over the body and energy awareness. The last four limbs work on the mind, senses and attaining a higher state of consciousness.

The sutras contain guidelines for correct living and ways to attain Kaivalya or liberation from the cycle of birth and death through the practice of meditation. Ashtanga or the 'eight limbs' of yoga are the guidance and steps towards the goal of liberation (from the restlessness of the mind).

1. **Yamas**
2. **Niyamas**
3. **Asanas**
4. **Pranayama**
5. **Pratyahara**
6. **Dharana**
7. **Dhyana**
8. **Samadhi**

LIMB 1: YAMAS
Guidelines for ethical standards and moral restraints, as listed by Patanjali.
They are subdivided into five different sections.

1. Ahimsa: non-violence, non-injury; consideration and compassion for all living beings including yourself.

Most modern yogis equate non-violence to vegetarianism, which is one aspect. This is a difficult path to follow, as many living creatures are harmed even when pulling the vegetables from the ground, so it is as near as impossible to 'do no harm' all the time. Every step we take has the possible action of harming insects and even the air we breathe contains microscopic life that we cannot avoid ingesting. The obvious non-harming of animals is a starting place.

Ahimsa is just as much about non-harming of yourself as well as animals or others. Telling yourself you have a 'bad back' or a 'bad knee' is in some ways using the power of the mind to tell yourself you are bad. The constant chit-chat of the mind that replays the past and predicts the future puts us through a mental disturbance that is essentially harmful as it stops us from living in the 'now'. If guilt plays a part in our lives at any point this too becomes harmful. For the things we cannot change, we must accept and move on. For the things we can change it is wise to try to sort it out so that the mind is allowed to alleviate any guilt and stop the self-punishment that the thoughts can bring.

2. **Satya:** truthfulness – non-telling of lies; living with honesty in behaviour, thought and intention.

Being honest with ourselves is possibly one of the most difficult things to do in life. Patanjali states within the sutras that living out from the heart centre causes pain. This pain will lead to dissatisfaction and this can lead to illness. In modern-day living many people are stuck in jobs, through circumstances of family and obligations, that stop them from living their true path. Some may say the true path is yoga, but for those who are yet to discover yoga it could simply be that they dreamed of being an artist or dancer but through life's circumstances their true existence and path has been diverted, leading them into a life that is not of their inner being. This can lead to subtle (often unknown, or unacknowledged) resentment, which in turn leads the inner beauty to be lost or displaced. All these subtle imbalances may be the cause of suffering, which in turn may lead to disease within the self, which could in time lead to the manifestation of illness. In the book *The Top Five Regrets of the Dying* by Bronnie Ware, a nurse who for 12 years took care of people during their final days of life, the number one regret was listed as 'I wish I'd had the courage to live a life true to myself, not the life others expected of me.'

3. **Asteya**: no stealing – no jealousy; cultivating a less materialistic view. Stop desiring what we may not have.

A deeper dimension of asteya is the theft of someone else's reputation through a negative opinion. In yoga we believe that every action has a reaction or consequence. When a yoga student asks 'have you heard of so-and-so's class, is she any good?' the answer you give would be, if negative (even though not done in malice), a stealing of someone's reputation. Yes, people may argue you are allowed to give your opinion, however, what one yoga practitioner gives in their teaching may not be your cup of tea but the person enquiring may find their teaching inspirational. This can be said of many different things in life: 'have you seen the latest Batman movie?', 'have you eaten in that restaurant?', and so on. Every time we give our own personal opinion we incur karma, for there will be a consequence of your comments. There are so many different styles of yoga class out there today (many of which are Hatha based) and there are many teachers who dismiss other styles for one reason or another (usually due to their passion for the style they fell in love with), however it is still a little disappointing that this happens even among yoga teachers. Non-stealing goes beyond shoplifting from a supermarket – it is so much deeper than that. Yoga is about being equal at all times, balanced and dispassionate in the aim of incurring no negative karma, and as opinions can have so many consequences, they are not worth giving.

4. **Brahmacharya:** moderation – chastity; non-indulgence of the senses. Not using sexuality and flirtatiousness for self-reward, ego, and or gain.

In the householder path (discussed in chapter 8) the meaning of Bramacharya means faithfulness to one's partner and loved ones. The Indriyas (senses) can, if uncontrolled, lead us to distractions of many kinds. The true householder yogi does not allow his senses to be drawn to those who have external beauty and therefore does not allow lust (which, according to *The Bhagavad Gita*, leads to greed and jealousy, and thus to the gates to hell), to become distracted or drawn in by individuals who live from their primal instinct of sex and sexuality. These individuals who use their powers of flirtatiousness and sex to get what they want in life are living a life that is the opposite of yoga. This also goes for the yoga teachers who thrive on the joy of class numbers being high and their own popularity. This only invigorates the ego and tells us we are the ones that people are practising yoga for, when really it should be your teachings and the light of yoga that draw people to your classes. The demonstration of complicated asanas and the wearing of body-hugging clothing can be seen by some as a way to overcome the yoga teachers desire to be liked as many students believe their teacher should have a great practice and physique. Those yoga swamis who renounce ego when teaching a Hatha yoga class very rarely demonstrate a single asana, instead they use their guidance to teach the postures, or ask a class member to demonstrate the asana for those who do not know how to do it.

5. **Aparigraha**: non-attachment – non-accepting of gifts; judge your success by who you are, not by what you have. Appreciate all that you have such as health, happiness, family, time, love, etc.

Non-attachment is a very difficult subject, especially if you have children. 'How can one not be attached to their child'? This is a very emotive subject, which can only be resolved by each individual. In the householder path of yoga, when one becomes a forest dweller and then sannyasin (monk) at the later stages of life, this is when all attachments are given up forever, including family. To know this would be your path would ensure that throughout your life you nurtured, enjoyed and taught your children everything possible to allow them to be successful in their own lives, and when the day of renunciation comes, you would feel blessed in knowing your progeny were developed, strong and beautiful human beings as you prepare for the next life. Non-attachment to material things is an easier subject to discuss, as in yoga there is a belief that what you hold onto in this life will be carried through to the next. Financial wealth is a wondrous thing if used for the good of others and to further your own spiritual practice. Those who have the opportunity to use their financial status to make time for their own self-development and to help out those less fortunate are indeed blessed. Those, however who choose to work endlessly to attain wealth for bigger and better material things are distracting themselves from the true goal of life, which is to attain spiritual bliss and to enjoy the things you have that money cannot buy, such as health, love, inner peace and happiness, all of which are achievable through yoga practices. Non-accepting of gifts is a subject that may seem hard to understand for some. Attachment to another person can come from accepting a gift from them. Some people may buy gifts for others and then call upon 'favours' in return. This attachment and obligation came about because the gift was accepted.

LIMB 2: NIYAMAS
Observances and disciplines; our attitude towards ourselves.

They are subdivided into five different sections.

1. **Saucha**: purity; physical, mental and environmental cleanliness. Saucha is a state of mental, physical and to some extent environmental cleanliness.

For the mind to be pure, the thought waves must be stilled to stop the chit-chat of the past and future stirring up one's mental state, which can in turn lead to thoughts that are impure, angry and useless. Physical cleanliness comes about through giving our bodies their essential nutritional needs. The over-indulgence of food and alcohol is an indication of emotional gratification that has been either embedded from childhood or caused by unhappiness in adult life.

Yoga can bring inner reflection and peace of mind that helps to purify and cleanse. The environmental cleanliness that the world needs is being ignored by many due to their lack of anything other than I-am awareness. The planet we live on works very hard to adapt to the exploitation of its natural resources. The more people who practise yoga and begin to live with love for all, the more we will stop destroying our natural habitat.

2. **Santosha**: contentment – a positive outlook and uncomplaining attitude. Santosha is at the very heart of yoga.

If we are content with what we have in life we do not look elsewhere for gratification. The ego, once controlled, allows us to be content and happy with our lives as they are. Seeing everything as perfect in our lives is a true sign of Santosha. Even when things seem like they are dark and heavy, everything in life is an opportunity to learn, and contentment helps us harness this learning to further encourage our spiritual growth.

3. **Tapas**: austerities – purifying practices. Self-control and discipline with enthusiasm for life.

In ancient times in India yogis were called Tapasvins as they would sit in austerity or discomfort in the practice of 'stewing in their own juices', (Feuerstein, 1998). This action of making themselves uncomfortable by whatever means would bring about a mind state that would be a whirlpool of darkness and distraction. In turn, the self-study from such dark and depressing thoughts would help them further their spiritual growth by acknowledging, accepting and releasing their deepest most unthinkable thoughts.

Very few people today verbalise their innermost thoughts. This could be due to society's vision of what is socially acceptable, and some might say these trapped and hidden thoughts can lead to mental illness and depression.

4. **Swadhyaya**: study of spiritual scriptures. Self-study, mindfulness, reflection and self-discovery.

After spending time listening to the chatter of the mind, self-study begins. It takes immense growth and strength to acknowledge our own need to expand and this is where self-study takes place. True yoga begins when we recognise our own faults and failings and work beyond them to improve ourselves, and to watch our emotions and thoughts control the habits that may occur from such inner awareness.

5. **Ishwara pranidhana**: surrender to God – practice of awareness, accepting there is a higher

force. Patanjali talks of Purusa and Prakruti (the two primordial forces of nature) and ways to attain God.

Without acceptance of a higher power there would be no reason to study the sutras and therefore it is a principle found within the Niyamas. It is considered that some yoga practitioners can begin their Hatha yoga journey without the practice of the Yamas and Niyamas and that through the daily routines of asanas, pranayama, mudra, bandhas, that the mind will eventually still to the point where the above guidance will naturally fall into place.

LIMB 3: ASANAS
Physical postures

For many, this is their starting point in yoga. The body is the temple of the spirit. Practice of asana brings discipline and concentration, both essential for meditation. Patanjali however does not prescribe more than three asanas, which are traditionally seated poses.

Patanjali states in the Yoga Sutras: Book 2 – Ways to attain yoga.

> 46 – Postures (asanas) should be steady and pleasant.
> 47 – Asanas are mastered by relaxed effort and remaining unaware of the body.
> 48 – From that, one is no longer disturbed by the dualities, hot/cold, pleasure/pain.
> (Prabhavananda and Isherwood, 1953).

LIMB 4: PRANAYAMA
Control of life force or energy done through breathing exercises

The practice of pranayama helps to gain mastery over the respiratory process, connecting the breath, the mind, and the emotions, and has many powerful effects on the whole being. See chapter 5 for further details.

LIMB 5: PRATYAHARA
Sensory detachment/withdrawal of the senses; control of the mind to focus within

This practice gives us a chance to step back and take a look at ourselves from within, to check and observe any habits and cravings, which may interfere with our spiritual growth. The withdrawal of the senses can help release us from our negative habits by removing the external distractions that result in the constant flitting of the mind.

LIMB 6: DHARANA
Concentrating the mind to the exclusion of all other thoughts; the path to the seventh and eighth limbs

Once Pratyahara is practised we can relieve ourselves from outside distractions and move onto the distractions of the mind itself. Dharana helps to slow down the thinking process by concentrating our thoughts to one point. Silent repetition of a sound, focusing on a deity or energy point in the body will help in long periods of concentration. This naturally leads us into Dhyana (meditation).

LIMB 7: DHYANA
Meditation or contemplation; an unbroken flow of thought inwards and thus to the higher self

Dhyana is the uninterrupted flow of concentration leading to the meditative state.

LIMB 8: SAMADHI
The enlightened state of bliss transcending the self and becoming one with the Supreme Consciousness

The ultimate goal of any human being is to find peace. During meditation the yogi joins with their point of focus and transcends the self altogether, relieving them from the afflictions of mortality by tapping into the cosmic forces. With this connection to the cosmic life force there comes an understanding of all living things and beyond. Meditation brings a state of bliss and being at one with the Universe. Enlightenment cannot be possessed or bought, it can only be experienced, and the price of this is discipline, (Sivananda, 1986).

> *According to The Yoga Sutras of Patanjali:*
> *– Attention leads to concentration (3.1)*
> *– Concentration leads to meditation (3.2)*
> *– Meditation leads to Samadhi (3.3).*
>   (Sivananda, 1986).

The final three limbs (Dharana, Dhyana, Samadhi) are collectively known as Samyama and are progressive stages of meditation. These collectively create a form of absorption within the object of focus, which is considered a point of enlightenment by 'becoming the object'. This 'becoming' through Samyama awakens our potential to other realities and knowledge, (Sivananda, 1986).

THE BHAGAVAD GITA, THE CELESTIAL SONG OR THE SONG OF THE LORD

At the heart of Indian culture is the story in myth, legend and religion of the Mahabharata. The first known written versions are estimated to date back to the fifth century BCE and are considered to be one of the world's oldest stories, fifteen times the length of the Bible.

The poem's authorship is commonly attributed to Vyasa, and it consists of over 100,000 verses, although volumes change with translations so this is not a definitive number. The subject of the poem is based on a war that probably happened around 1500 BCE. It explores the heights and depths of the human soul and psyche, illustrating in dramatic form how good Hindus should live their lives. It is universally renowned as the jewel of India's spiritual wisdom. Embedded in book six of the Mahabharata is *The Bhagavad Gita* (Song of the Lord), a mystical poem about life, death, love, and duty.

The central story is of the lifelong feud between two families, the Pandavas (the 'good' guys) and the Kauravas (the 'bad' guys), two closely related regal families, and the final battle which will decide once and for all which family will be supreme.

The opening of the Gita is at the beginning of the great battle between the two families and involves a dialogue between Arjuna, who is considered the great hero and his charioteer, who is Krishna incarnated to bring the message to the world. Arjuna is faced with the dilemma of whether he should fight or not.

Arjuna is overcome with anguish when he sees in the opposing army many of his kinsmen, teachers, and friends. Tens of thousands of good men were about to die, leaving a generation to grow up without fathers. It would take decades for the kingdom to recover from the staggering losses about to ensue. He does not want to fight and turns to his charioteer for advice.

Should Arjuna conform to his duty as a warrior and fight, and in so doing kill the people fighting for his enemy who are also his teachers, kinsmen and friends? Or, should he refuse to join the battle and disrupt the natural order? To take either path would seem to bring bad results for all.

Since his charioteer is God in the form of Krishna, the advice takes the form of spiritual teachings on the different paths of yoga, teaching him the real nature of action (*karma*) and its effects. It is considered Krishna incarnated from his original form as Vishnu to bring this knowledge of righteousness or Dharma to mankind to remind them of the ways to live a good life.

Action performed disinterestedly, without attachment to the results (Karma yoga), has no bad effects for the person. According to this compromise, one should perform one's inherent duty, that is, conform to one's 'social' role – but renounce internally.

In fact, Krishna, who reveals himself thus to be God, the omnipotent maintainer and destroyer of the universe, acts at the universal level in precisely this way himself. By activating his lower or material nature, he has brought the universe into being, but he observes his creation dispassionately.

Krishna reveals to Arjuna that the individual soul (atman) is eternal and indestructible: it neither kills nor is killed, and is identical with the absolute power (Brahman) underlying all phenomena. Krishna advises Arjuna to fight, but without attachment for the end result. This will free him from the three qualities of nature also known as the three gunas, (Feuerstein, 1998). These are introduced over the page.

The Gita teaches us about Dharma which is the best possible course, or righteousness, the fulfillment of one's true purpose or virtue (connected to caste and social status).

THE VISION OF GOD

Arjuna knows Krishna is God in disguise and wants to see what God really looks like. So once Arjuna agrees to fight he asks Krishna for a favour and asks him to reveal his true self to him, and so Krishna shows him. Arjuna sees universes without end, galaxies spinning in and out of existence. He sees trillions and trillions of souls trapped in the cycle of birth and death, being born, suffering, dying and being reborn again over and over. For a mind that has not yet been completely purified by spiritual practice, the vision is too much to bear. Arjuna begs for Krishna to stop and the Lord resumes his human form, (Feuerstein, 1998).

THE MAIN DOCTRINES OF THE GITA

- **Karma yoga**: the yoga of selfless action performed with inner detachment from its results
- **Bhakti yoga**: the yoga of devotion to a particular god – in this case Krishna
- **Jnana yoga**: the yoga of knowledge and discrimination between the lower nature of man and his soul through study
- **Raja yoga**: the yoga of meditation.

THE THREE GUNAS

The Gita also introduces the three gunas, natures or qualities. These are:
1. **Sattva**: purity and knowledge, in food, thought and heart
2. **Rajas**: activity and motion, in daily life and mindfulness
3. **Tamas**: laziness and poison, it is also the guna that allows us to sleep, for without inertia we would never be able to rest.

Together the three gunas (or qualities) are balanced within every aspect of nature. A person will have all three qualities within themselves, with one quality predominant at any given moment. A person may be very sattvic in nature (relaxed, chilled out, unfazed by most things) but may become rajasic (excited and passionate) when something stimulates them. Another person may be very rajasic most of the time and then become sattvic at the end of a busy and demanding day when they return home and calm the mind.

The yogi's duty is to try to stay sattvic, eat sattvic and think/live a sattvic life. The householder yogi allows the rajasic side to be removed through householder duties such as work and yoga asana, compared to the sannyasin that remains sattvic even during work. All three gunas are important in maintaining a balanced life, (Lad, 2002).

THE FOUR BASIC URGES AND THE FOUR STAGES OF LIFE (ASHRAMAS)

The ancient seers observed that mankind has four basic urges. These urges are:
- **Dharma**: right living and thinking
- **Artha**: the acquisition of wealth through honest means
- **Kama**: pleasurable experiences in life
- **Moksha**: the fulfilment of spiritual liberation.

The great sages then prescribed four stages of life in order to allow people to accomplish the four basic urges, which they then prescribed into a four-fold pathway, known as:

The four ashramas
- **Brahmacharya**: the first stage is the life of a celibate disciplined student devoted to moral and knowledgeable truths
- **Grahastya**: the second stage is that of married life where one works and has a family, this is known as the householder stage
- **Vanaprastha**: the stage once known as the 'forest dweller stage', where the householder passes on his/her material wealth and worldly affairs to his children while acting as counsel for their guidance and yet at the same time begins a more spiritual inward practice in preparation for the final stage
- **Sannyasin**: the fourth and final stage is living the life of a monk, renouncing the world completely in favour of devotion and service to God, in preparation for the next life, (Chanchani and Chanchani, 1995).

THE BODY AND MIND ACCORDING TO YOGA

THE BODY ACCORDING TO YOGA

In the modern Western world, the physical body (anatomical and physiological structures and systems), material world (possessions and objects) and scientific method (quantitative information and evidence-based practice) are most people's focus for reality and existence. These physical and material concepts are things that can be experienced by the physical body and the senses (sight, sound, taste etc.) and understood by the rational mind.

In Eastern philosophies (yoga, Chinese medicine and martial arts etc.) and many other philosophies (Celtic, Pagan etc.), beliefs extend beyond the physical and material realms and towards the spiritual dimensions, and the existence of alternative energy forces in the cosmos, for example: ki, qi or chi (Taoist) and prana (Hindu), aether (alchemy), ka (Egyptian), mahan (Australian Aboriginal).

Historically, the West and some religions have discouraged belief and discussion of these energy forces, believing them to be dangerous, (Bloom, 2011:203). Spiritual and energetic teachings have often been excluded from some yoga and martial arts practice, and taught only to trusted students because of this. However, more recently there has been an increasing interest and awareness of these alternative forces. There is a greater acceptance that the material and physical world is just one aspect to existence and there is also a growing awareness and belief that individuals and groups can consciously and unconsciously affect the world through their thoughts and energy vibrations, (Bloom, 2011:204).

THE THREE BODIES (SHARIRA) ACCORDING TO YOGA

Many different yoga scriptures describe each person as made up of three bodies: physical, energetic and subtle (see figure 2.1). These three bodies are where our form, energy and imprint of 'who we are' come together at a specific point during growth in the womb and at birth. The chanting of the three Oms at the beginning or ending of any spiritual practice or yoga class is done to purify each body.

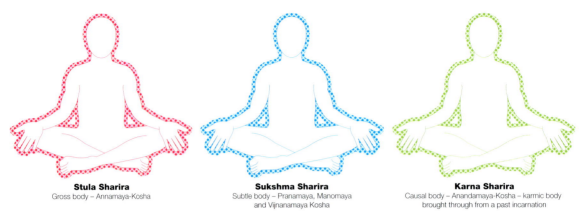

Figure 2.1 Sharira Treeni (The three bodies)

PRANA AND THE 'ENERGETIC' BODY

Yoga is often called the science of self realization, because its end result is a realization of just who we are, not limiting that knowledge to our surface personality, or the ego-led persona that we project out into the world, but discovering the real person, the self hidden deep inside, which yoga declares to be spirit itself.

(Forstater and Manuel, 2002:15)

The Panch Maya Koshas (energy bodies/layers)

In yogic physiology, there are five (some texts say seven) sheaths/illusions (kosa or koshas) that represent different layers of existence and correspond with different states of consciousness. These layers were offered by the ancient sages as a way to help man understand himself, (Iyengar, 1996:51 and 141). In the West, they may be known as auras.

These include:
- **Annamaya kosha**: the anatomical or material body (earth)
- **Pranamaya kosha**: the physiological, energy, bioplasmic and lifeforce body (water)
- **Manomaya kosha**: the mental or psychological body (fire)
- **Vijnamaya kosha**: the psychic or higher mental or intellectual body (air)
- **Anandamaya kosha**: the transcendental or bliss body (ether).

NB: Some texts also reference two additional sheaths, (Iyengar, 1996:141):
- **Cittamaya kosha**: the consciousness body (celestial)
- **Atmamaya kosha**: the self body (luminous).

The energy bodies or sheaths represent different layers of consciousness and an individual's vibration (see figure 2.2). Table 2.1 describes the different energy bodies.

Each of the five layers are frontiers which need to be understood and integrated between the *seen*, the material (prakriti) and the *seer*, perceiver (purusa). That is, integration of the body, the senses, energy, mind, intellect, consciousness and soul and with consideration to the corresponding different levels of consciousness (citta) or awareness, (Iyengar, 1993:137).

The aspirant (through yoga practice) conquers his body, controls his energy, restrains the mind, develops sound judgement, from which he acts rightfully and becomes luminous; developing total awareness of his core being, achieves supreme knowledge and surrenders himself to the Supreme soul, universal self, (Paramatman).

B.K.S. Iyengar, (1993:139)

Understanding and using the five sheaths

Although many people understand the concept of the five sheaths, it is, for some, a huge leap of faith to truly believe they exist. After spending ten days at the Sivananda Ashram Austria, studying the Yoga of the Heart (a teacher training course taught by Nischala Joy Devi for yoga for cancer and life-threatening illnesses), Conrad Paul connected with the meaning and understanding of the koshas. The koshas are in order from physical to blissful for a reason and are considered layers of 'energy', which correlate to a different and specific 'energy' of the human being, with each one becoming more difficult to access except with continuous and dedicated yoga practice (of several decades). Through many years of effort, Samadhi or Bliss can be achieved using the anandamaya kosha and the sheaths before it. For most people the activation of the early sheaths is the first step.

1. Annamaya kosha: the physical sheath (physical body)

The easiest layer to access is the physical sheath and it is the layer everyone accesses every day without actual conscious connection. As the body is dense it is easy to understand that this body is the most gross or heavy with self-awareness and I-am-ness, which creates an illusion of a physical body. The energy built up in this body is used to make asanas as well as everyday activities. When the second sheath (life-force sheath) is properly activated the physical body has life, energy and relatively good health. Good living, right thought and regular asana practice helps to keep this energy vibrant and flowing. Bad habits, loss of practice and negative thinking will result in a waste of energy, which leaves the body drained and sluggish.

2. Pranamaya kosha: the life force sheath (pranic body)

This sheath is activated by the practice of 'full yogic breath' (see page 153) while lying perfectly still and relaxed. The deep breathing fully revitalises the energy sheath and the stillness of the body allows the life force to build. After five minutes the energy levels have built sufficiently

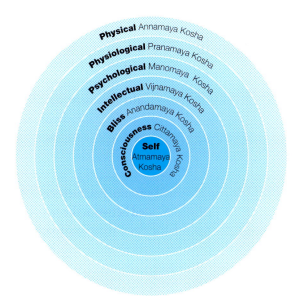

Figure 2.2 The Koshas or body sheaths

to become a useful boost for the first sheath, annamaya kosha, so it can perform asanas and daily activities with full intent and without effort. Intentionally sending the energy into the physical sheath allows the practice of daily life with joy and ease. If the energy is sent into the third sheath (manomaya kosha, the mind energy sheath), then the built-up energy can be used in a different way for health and well-being. After activating the second sheath the energy built up is sent into the mind energy for efficient and powerful use. Many believe in mind over matter, (Lipton, 2005).

3. **Manomaya kosha – the mind sheath (mind body)**

The mind body or sheath is one of the most powerful sheaths to activate due to the mind's power over the body, (Lipton, 2005). Once the pranamaya kosha has been charged, if the aspirant lies still, the built-up energy can be drawn into the mind sheath, which then has a super-charged effect on the body. Harnessing the power of the mind in healing is part of an ancient yoga and ayurveda tradition and has shown to help people recovering from major illnesses when all hope was lost and conventional medicine had ceased its intervention, (Tiwari, 1995). Major studies in America on cancer care and heart disease recovery have shown that deep relaxation and positive thinking as part of a programme of well-being for those suffering from a life-threatening illness often has life-extending consequences, (Ornish *et al*, 2005). The positive aspect of the mind can be scientifically proven to be beneficial, and ancient yoga techniques show us the way to fully use this tool for healing and happiness, (Lipton, 2005).

> ### Annamaya kosha activation: initial relaxation
>
> **Physical body utilisation**
>
> Relaxed breathing, bring awareness to and relax your:
> - feet, ankles, calves, shins, knees, thighs, buttocks, hips and pelvis
> - fingers, hands, wrists, forearms, elbows, upper arms, shoulders, shoulder sockets
> - lower back and abdomen, middle back and chest, upper back and clavicles, armpits
> - neck, throat, head and face, eyes, nose, cheeks, jaw and mouth, tongue and teeth
> - brain, heart, lungs, digestive system, kidneys, liver.
>
> Picture your mind still and calm.
>
> The body is now ready to receive energy or relaxation.

Prana (absolute energy)

Prana is a key concept in Ayurvedic medicine and yoga. The word prana evolves from Sanskrit and translates as 'breath' or 'absolute energy' or 'go everywhere'. Prana is the life force that flows through all things and is contained in food, water and thoughts. Prana is at the heart of all yoga practice, that is, through the practice of breathing (pranyama) and asanas (postures), as well as other techniques. Through practising these techniques, the individual generates more prana and vitality.

Life force or prana is the elementary precept of vayu (air). It is the fundamental energy that enters the being at birth and departs at the end of life, and connects the mind, body and spirit. It flows through, and to, every cell in the body, and without

> **Pranamaya kosha activation: full yogic breath**
>
> Energy body utilisation
> Begin to bring awareness to your breathing.
> - Inhale into abdomen
> - Abdomen and chest
> - Abdomen, chest and collar bones
> - Reverse the breathing from clavicles, chest to abdomen.
>
> Focus on this for five minutes to activate the pranamaya kosha.
>
> The pranic sheath is now fully activated. It is up to the participant to send it either to the physical body or the mind, in what is known as the pranic sandwich.
>
> Send the energy built up here to the physical body and get up with new-found vigour.
>
> Send the energy into the manomaya kosha to utilise positive thinking for health and vitality.

> **Manomaya kosha activation: mind/body connection**
>
> Mind/body utilisation
> - Relax your breathing and as you gently inhale attach the breath to the mind and take it into the toes, as you exhale imagine the breath evaporating from the toes into the room as a golden light
> - Inhale, follow the mind and breath into the feet…
> - … and up the whole body, part by part
> - Once you have covered the internal organs, bring your thoughts to your heart centre and imagine a tiny flame flickering in your heart, as you inhale the flame grows brighter to fill the body, over time, with golden light
> - Finish by allowing yourself to come back to the room and wiggle the fingers and toes to awaken the physical sheath.

it life cannot continue, (Athique, 2009). Prana (life force) is supplied by the air that is breathed (oxygen), food, water, solar energy, and is taken up by the nervous system, (Sivananda, 1964). It manifests its subtle form into five divisions, within the pranamaya kosha. The five major pranas are known as panchas.

1. **Prana**: the first division is the vital air that enters the cell via the blood and is the essential force for all creation. It is the area between the larynx and the top of the diaphragm and is associated with all the muscles and nerves that activate speech and respiration. It also controls the oesophagus.

2. **Apana**: is the release into the bloodstream of carbon wastes, and is the prana of elimination and detoxification. It is located below the navel and provides energy for the kidneys, liver, intestines and genitals.

3. **Samana**: governs the balance between prana and apana in the cells, as it is the equalising force of the Universe. It is located between the heart and the navel and activates the digestive system (stomach, pancreas, intestines, liver, etc.) and their secretions.

4. **Udana**: is the chemical message transmitted between the cells, and is the force of creative expression and upward movement. It controls the area above the neck and activates the sensory receptors (eyes etc.) and activates the limbs and associated tissues (joints, muscles, ligaments, nerves), harmonising movement and posture.

Table 2.1	The energy bodies and koshas
Physical or material body **Anatomical sheath** **Annamaya kosha**	The anatomical and physical body, which we attribute as being part of ourselves. The muscular and skeletal system (bones and joints), circulatory and respiratory system, nervous system, digestive system etc. Cleansed through asana practice and appropriate diet and nutrition.
Astral or emotional **Physiological/lifeforce sheath** **Pranamaya kosha**	The astral body carries emotions, feelings and personality traits. The aura of the astral body can extend a few metres beyond the sphere of the physical body and reflects the emotional state by displaying different colours (visible to some, invisible to most). The astral or emotional body is in constant motion, mirroring all feelings and thoughts as they flow through awareness (conscious or unconscious). It stores all unresolved issues (fears of loneliness, abandonment, rejection) etc. The energy vibrations held in this body radiate out and often attract others with the same vibrations and who mirror the unconscious or sub-conscious aspects of ourselves. It is believed these unresolved issues and emotions are carried forward into, and create, different incarnations. Emotional knots manifest in the solar plexus centre (chakra) and if the individual is ready to confront these issues, the third eye chakra can be used to explore these. However, resolution of the issues comes from the higher-self aspect and the engagement of the heart and crown chakra, to regard all experiences with a sense of empathy, acceptance and non-judgement. It is believed that when we experience ourself as a victim in this lifetime, we were a persecutor in a previous incarnation. Being able to observe all the unusual visions, sensations and images that may present through this body, with no judgement, enables the opportunity to heal. The more healing that takes place, the more the astral body radiates a clear and bright glow reflecting (and attracting) love and happiness. Pranamaya kosha is made up of five major pranas, collectively known as pancha: • Prana vayu – located in the chest and deals with respiration • Apana vayu – located in the abdomen and deals with elimination/excretion • Samana vayu – located in the middle of the body, the fire centre, digestion • Udana – located in the head and deals with thought and expression/speech • Vyana – deals with the whole body, circulation and all life processes. Cleansed through pranayama (breathing) – see chapter 5

Table 2.1 The energy bodies and koshas, continued

Mental/Ethereal **Psychological sheath** **Manomaya kosha**	The mental body (aura) draws on the energy from the chakras and nadis and passes this energy to the physical body. This layer provides protection against external energies that may contribute to illness. Negative behaviours (excessive use of alcohol or nicotine, poor diet, negative thoughts) lower the energy vibration of the ethereal body and create weak areas or holes that allow positive energies to escape and negative energies to be taken in. Energy can be restored in this body by spending time in natural environments and close to plants, flowers, water, fields and nature e.g. lying down on the grass or hugging a tree. Cleansed through the practice of yamas, niyamas and selfless service (Karma Path).
Intellectual/wisdom **Intellectual sheath** **Vijnamaya kosha**	The intellectual body aura extends beyond both the physical and astral body. All thoughts, ideas, intuitions are reflected in the intellectual body. The more open one's thoughts and the deeper the awareness, the brighter and clearer will be the colours vibrated in this aura. Alternatively, narrow and linear thinking will dull the vibrations in this aura. The intellectual body and the quality of our thoughts are affected by the feelings of the emotional body; therefore to some extent, thinking is always 'clouded' (despite the belief that rational thinking exists). Connecting with the third eye and crown chakras enables 'rational' thoughts to be viewed in light with the higher aspect of self. There is greater connection with wisdom and universal spiritual truths, which may reveal themselves as insights or sound (which may include hearing voices or seeing visions). Cleansed through meditation, appropriate enquiry (who am I?) and reading of the ancient scriptures.
Spiritual **The sheath of bliss** **Anandamaya kosha**	The spiritual body vibrates at a higher frequency than the other energy bodies and reflects an enlightened state of being and a connection with all things. An openness to the vibrations of this energy body allows all actions to come from a place of compassion, wisdom and bliss – the higher self. Cleansed through Samadhi. This is the most important of the sheaths and is reached through the practice of Raja yoga.

5. **Vyana**: the distribution through the cell of vital energy; it is the external circulating power of the cosmos, (Beal, 2011). It balances, coordinates and acts as a reserve energy source for all other pranas (as above).

All cells within the human body have an individual as well as a collective role, integrating with other cells to perpetuate unified balance. Science shows us that stem cells become specialised in a series of events known as cell differentiation, where they are given individual tasks, or made self aware, which is part of a cooperative to maintain physical life, (Waugh & Grant (2010). The order and intellect of the body's cells is considered to be formed of supreme intelligence known as Mahad. Cellular intelligence, and communication between cells is achieved through the transmitted flow of this Universal energy or prana, (Lad, 2002).

The frequency at which prana is generated, absorbed and stored, determines the individual's level of consciousness and the degree of connectedness between the astral and physical bodies.

Lifestyle has a profound impact on prana and the flow of energy. Energy and prana will be affected by the intake of food, exercise and activity, sexual behaviour, thinking patterns (stress etc.) and relationships with others. Any imbalance will be felt and experienced as being drained of energy, which in turn, can affect the health of specific organs and may impact their functioning.

Pranayama and breathwork (chapter 4) have a vital role to play in maintaining health. Most people have developed a pattern of short, shallow breathing, using only part of the lungs. Yoga practice helps to bring the breath under more conscious control and encourages more effective breathing patterns, which help to restore energy and balance and bring stillness and clarity to the mind.

It is believed that prana flows through invisible channels referred to as nadis (discussed below). Prana gives the body life for the time the soul abides within the body. When the body dies, prana, the life force leaves the body.

NADIS

Techniques used to cleanse the nadis are pranayama (chapter 4) and the kriyas (chapter 6) and asanas (chapter 4). The term 'nadi' means 'flow', 'current', 'pipe' (Fig 2.3) or 'vessel'. Energy or prana flows through these invisible channels. If the nadis are blocked, then prana will also be restricted which can result in a lack of energy and poor health.

It is estimated that there are 72,000 nadis, (Sharamon and Baginski 1991), although some texts indicate that there are three or four times this number. In Chinese medicine, a similar system of channels are the meridians. The main nadis include: ida, pingala and sushumna (see table 2.2).

CHAKRAS

The aim of yoga is the union of Goddess Shakti (kundalini energy, which awakens in the root chakra) and the joining of this with God Shiva (supreme consciousness, which resides in the crown chakra).

Shakti ascends through sushumna, passing through the chakras. When Shakti unites with ida (yin, cooling, moon energy, feminine) and pingala (yang, warming, sun energy, masculine) in the Ajna Chakra, this is Hatha Yoga (the first union); when Shakti reaches the crown chakra and unites with Shiva, this is yoga (the ultimate union).

Hatha Yoga Pradipka 1993:13.
Swami Muktibodhananda

Table 2.2 Main Nadis

Ida	Left side of body Moon/night Feminine Cooling energy Yin Dark Subconscious mind Parasympathetic nervous system Desire
Pingala	Right side of body Sun/day Masculine Warming energy Yang Light Conscious mind Sympathetic nervous system Action
Sushumna	Central – through the spine from the coccyx to the crown of the head and through the corresponding chakras (root to crown) Cosmic light Androgynous Temperate Tao Unconscious mind Central nervous system Knowledge Kundalini rises from the root chakra at the base of the sushumna, increasing consciousness (Kundalini is awakened by yoga practices, which include pranayama) Shiva (the destroyer of ignorance) flows down from the crown chakra to build supreme consciousness

Adapted from: Sharamon, S. & Baginski, B. (1997) & Swami Muktibodhananda (HYP, 1993)

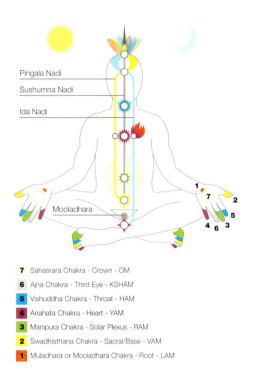

7 Sahasrara Chakra - Crown - OM
6 Ajna Chakra - Third Eye - KSHAM
5 Vishuddha Chakra - Throat - HAM
4 Anahata Chakra - Heart - YAM
3 Manipura Chakra - Solar Plexus - RAM
2 Swadhisthana Chakra - Sacral/Base - VAM
1 Muladhara or Mooladhara Chakra - Root - LAM

Figure 2.3 Chakra Sapta (The seven chakras)

In Sanskrit, the word chakra, means 'ring', 'circle' or 'wheel'. However, a more fitting translation may be 'vortex' or 'whirlpool'.

The seven main chakras (see figure 2.4) are invisible energy centres that are positioned along the length of the spine, from the crown of the head to the tailbone. It is believed they govern all elements of the body, hold aspects of our energy and determine the energetic wellness of the body and mind. The chakras connect to the nadis or energy channels (ida, pingala and sushumna) and move prana (the life force) through these channels and transmit cosmic energy into spiritual energy.

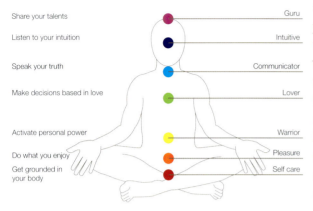

Figure 2.4 Chakras and attributes

It is believed that in most people the chakras are inactive and lay dormant. The aim of yoga practice is to awaken the energy in the chakras through the practice of asana and pranayama, which activates the nadis, causing the chakras to vibrate and release their coiled-up energy. Concentration on the specific chakras during asana practice (and/or during meditation) helps to activate them and stimulate the flow of spiritual energy to reach higher levels of consciousness. The chakras are believed to be accessible once the student has accomplished the right limbs of practice, discussed earlier, (BKS Iyengar, 2001.36).

Self-realisation is achieved through practice. When the devoted student or aspirant learns to release anger, desire, greed, infatuation, pride and envy (avidya), which are blocks to contentment and happiness, they reach the bliss state. Some modern approaches to energy and healing work, suggest that chakra therapy and healing can begin before this, as it is one of the more gentle healing approaches.

Ida represents the negative force, the flow of consciousness; pingala represents the positive force, the flow of vital energy; and sushumna represents the neutral force, the spiritual energy.

HYP 1993:12, Swami Muktibodhananda

The connections of the chakras can be likened to the connection of the central nervous system with the peripheral nervous system; however, their effect is spiritual, rather than physiological.

When kundalini energy is awakened in the root chakra (muladhara) it rises upwards through the other chakras. The union with the nadis (ida and pingala) at ajna (third eye) chakra is Hatha yoga. The union with the crown chakra (sahasara) is the ultimate union of yoga (rather than Hatha yoga). Yoga is the union of shiva (supreme consciousness) and shakti (kundalini energy). Shiva flows down through the crown, to destroy ignorance or avidya.

GRANTHIS

Granthis are knots or blockages to pranic/psychic energy in the body. The granthis prevent the free flow of prana along sushumna nadi and impede the awakening of the chakras and the rising of the kundalini until such times that the individual is ready. They act like circuit breakers to stop the flow of energy/prana, preventing energy overload, which it is believed can be potentially harmful. Through proper guidance, right living and meditation the granthis are dissolved at the right and safe time; at which point they will be pierced by the movement of prana.

The granthis represent three levels of psychophysical life:
- The first knot (Brahma Granthi) is below the navel (muldahara or root chakra). When the flow of energy is restricted to this region, instinctive drives like hunger, thirst and sensory pleasure dominate the mind.
Attachment to desires. This granthi needs to be open and purified before kundalini will rise higher.
- The second knot (Vishnu Granthi) is below the heart (anahata or heart chakra). This is the region of the emotional life of the human being.
Attachment to actions. This granthi needs to be open and purified to allow kundalini energy to rise higher.
- The third knot (Rudra Granthi) is below the eyebrows (ajna – third eye chakra). This is the area of intellectual activity.
Attachment to thoughts. This granthi needs to be open and purified to allow kundalini energy to rise and connect with the crown chakra – for the ultimate union of Shakti and Shiva.

KUNDALINI

The concept of kundalini is one that is open to interpretation and misinterpretation. Translations and mistranslations of the ancient texts have led to some confusion, regarding how it is described and reported. It is suggested that even the *Hatha Yoga Pradipika* contains some contradictory explanations, (Desikachar, 1999:139).

In some teachings, Kundalini is described as the cosmic energy (the Goddess Shakti) believed to be dormant within everyone. Another term that has been used to describe this is agni (fire). Kundalini is often pictured as a coiled serpent lying at the base of the spine. The three main coils represent the three stages of the mind (avastha), which are: awake (jagrt), dreaming (svapna) and deep sleep (sushupti). The fourth stage, and final half coil is turiya, which is achived at enlightenment (Samadhi). Through a series of exercises involving posture, meditation, and breathing, a practitioner can awaken and release this energy up through the main channels (nadis and chakras) along the spine to the top of the head. This brings about a sensation of bliss, as the ordinary self is dissolved into its eternal essence: atman. When kundalini rises, it pierces the granthis and leads to liberation.

In some schools and traditions, kundalini energy is believed to be very powerful and thus should only be manipulated under the personal guidance of an experienced teacher. Other texts suggest that awakening kundalini can contribute to some experiences that many may find unusual and sometimes scary, including mental symptoms (psychosis – hearing voices, past life recall or paranoia) or physical symptoms (pain in the spine, muscle spasms, pressure in the third eye or crown chakra etc.) experienced when there is greater stored tension in the mind and body. However, meditation is believed to be the road through these experiences and can help to release these accumulated tensions, (Raven, 2000:56).

In other traditions kundalini is believed to be a metaphor for avidya or ignorance which is an obstacle to liberation. It is not believed to be a cosmic energy, as prana is the life force or energy and some authors suggest there cannot be two life forces, (Desikachar, 1999:139).

Table 2.3

Chakra name, meaning and mantra	Description	When functioning harmoniously (chakra open, energy uncoiled)	When functioning disharmoniously (chakra blocked, energy coiled) and associated developmental age
Seventh Sahasrara or crown chakra (Sahasrara means one thousand) Purest being. The gateway of the life-force – prana. **Mantra**: OM **Colours**: Violet, White, Gold	**Symbol**: 1,000 petalled shining lotus **Position**: At the top of the head. **Rotation**: Male – clockwise Female – anti-clockwise **Crystals**: Amethyst, rock crystal, diamond	Associated with deep thought. Developed sense of freedom. Inspiration and trust in life. A feeling of wholeness and abundance. The goal of all yoga. Uncoiled through intuitive knowledge. Being at one with the spiritual self, enlightenment. All ignorance is destroyed. There is courage, values and ethics. Increasing moments of bliss.	**Emotional and mental needs**: Separateness, fear and disconnection from wholeness and abundance. Prevents blockages in other chakras from being fully released. **Physical dysfunctions**: exhaustion, energetic disorders, mystical depression, confusion, Alzheimer's. **Hormonal connection**: Serotonin
Sixth Ajna or third eye chakra (Ajna means command) Knowledge of being **Mantra**: Ksham **Colours**: Indigo, yellow or violet	**Symbol**: 96 petalled silver lotus, 2 x 48 petals **Position**: Third eye, between the eyebrows **Guna**: Sattva **Rotation**: Male – anti-clockwise Female – clockwise **Crystals**: Lapis lazuli, indigo sapphire, amethyst, diamond	Associated with psychic ability and second sight. Developed humanity and spirituality. The mind is balanced and open to one's psychic nature, intuition, insight and mystic truths. There is clear vision. Non-judgemental self-awareness, feelings of adequacy and being enough, emotional intelligence, openness to the ideas of others.	**Emotional and mental needs**: Over-developed intellect. Arrogance, pride and desire. Inability to reflect spiritually or see the holistic nature of life and experiences, often unresolved emotional patterns. Muddled thinking, confusion, forgetfulness. **Physical dysfunctions**: Poor eyesight or hearing, seizures, conditions linked with the brain, spine and neurological connections, headaches, nightmares, hallucinations. **Hormonal connection**: Vasopressin (anti-diuretic)
Fifth Vishuditha chakra or throat chakra (Va means enhances; Shuddhi means purification) Resonance of being. **Mantra**: Ham **Colours**: Pale blue, silver, greenish blue	**Symbol**: 16 petalled violet lotus **Position**: Behind the throat **Guna**: Sattva **Rotation**: Male – clockwise Female – anti-clockwise **Crystals**: Aquamarine, turquoise, lapis lazuli, blue sapphire	Associated with communication. Self-determined. Able to express feelings, thoughts, inner knowledge and reveal strengths and weaknesses without fear. Personal expression, able to speak up for self, clear and imaginative speech, able to be silent and listen fully, able to say 'NO'.	**Emotional and mental needs**: Inability to openly express deepest truths and congruent feelings, for fear of judgement (self and others). Unable to show weakness. Not trusting of own intuition, blocked creativity. **Physical dysfunctions**: throat and mouth conditions, ulcers, swollen glands, gum problems, asthma, colds, stiff necks. **Hormonal connection**: Thyroxine **Developmental age**: 28–35
Fourth Anahata or heart chakra Devotion, self abandon	**Symbol**: 12 petalled blue lotus **Position**: Behind the sternum, level with heart	Associated with compassion, love and forgiveness. Developed compassion, spirituality and knowledge. Able to radiate warmth, sincerity, joy and unconditional love.	**Emotional and mental needs**: Expect gratitude and/or recognition for everything given. Unable to receive and accept love. Embarrassed by tenderness. Dependent on others for love.

Table 2.3 continued

Mantra: Yam **Colours**: Green, pink or gold	**Guna**: Rajas **Rotation**: Male – anti-clockwise Female – clockwise **Crystals**: Emerald, rose quartz, green jade, pink tourmaline	Put the heart into everything and give self freely, without expecting to gain.	**Physical dysfunctions**: heart and respiratory conditions, upper back and shoulder problems, high blood pressure, cancer. **Hormonal connection**: Thymus **Developmental age**: 21–28
Third Manipura or solar plexus chakra Shaping of being. **Mantra**: Ram **Colours**: Yellow or golden	**Symbol**: 10 petalled bright yellow lotus **Position**: Solar plexus or navel **Guna**: Rajas **Rotation**: Male – clockwise Female – anti-clockwise **Crystals**: Tiger's eye, citrine, yellow topaz	Associated with personal power – the body's stronghold. Calm with a sense of personal power. Acceptance and respect for both self and others. Able to integrate thoughts, feelings and wishes and develop a sense of wholeness. Strong sense of self and ability to make changes to self and life circumstances.	**Emotional and mental needs**: Fear and trust issues (the fear centre), a need to control and exercise power. Sensitivity to criticism, low self-esteem. Feel inadequate, easily upset and agitated, bottled up anger, sense of struggling to survive. **Physical dysfunctions**: gastrointestinal problems, arthritis, eating disorders, kidney or liver problems, chronic fatigue syndrome, stomach ulcers. **Hormonal connection**: Insulin **Developmental age**: 14–21
Second Swadhistana or base/sacral chakra (Swa means self; Sthan means dwelling) Creative reproduction of being. **Mantra**: Vam **Colour**: Orange	**Symbol**: 6 petalled crimson lotus **Position**: Two fingers higher than first chakra **Guna**: Tamas **Rotation**: Male – anti-clockwise Female – clockwise **Crystals**: Carnelian, moonstone, amber	Associated with emotions, intimacy and sensuality. Able to experience pleasure, and channel primal energy. Openness, ethics, honour and flow in personal relationships. Feelings are genuine and undistorted. Creativity, intimacy and sensuality. Ability to be flexible and flow. Ability to challenge motivations formed by social conditioning.	**Emotional and mental needs**: Influenced by worldly desires (money, sex, control and power). Inhibited expression. Sensual and sexual feelings held back (frigidity or impotence). Tendency to blame, feelings of guilt. **Physical dysfunctions**: Low back pain, sciatica, urinary problems, gynaecological problems. **Hormonal connection**: Oestrogen & testosterone **Developmental age**: 8–14
First Muladhara or Mooladhara or root (coccyx) chakra (Mool means root; Adhara means place) Physical will of being. The foundation and seat of all energy – kundalini. **Mantra**: Lam **Colour**: Fiery red	**Symbol**: 4 petalled deep red lotus **Position**: Perineum for men; cervix for women **Guna**: Tamas **Rotation**: Male – clockwise Female – anti-clockwise **Crystals**: Bloodstone, garnet, ruby, red coral, agate	Associated with sex drive and survival. Able to experience a deep sense of connection and relationship with the physical body and all earthly beings and creatures. Acceptance and gratitude for life and physical existence. Know their life path. The seat of the collective unconscious is accessible through this chakra.	**Emotional and mental needs**: Obsession with security, material possessions or sensual indulgences. Life experienced as a burden. Inability to let go or give or take freely. Incapable of inner stillness. **Physical dysfunctions**: Sciatica, low back pain, varicose veins, depression, constipation. **Hormonal connection**: Adrenaline & nor-adrenaline **Developmental age**: 1–8

Adapted from: Sharamon & Baginski (1997), Myss (1997), Raven (2000) & Swami Saradananda (2010)

Table 2.4 General overview of the Doshas

Dosha	Vata	Pitta	Kapha
First impressions	Unpredictable – Fast.	Intense – Fiery.	Relaxed – Slow.
Associated elements	Air and Space.	Fire and Water.	Earth and Water.
Qualities manifest as:	Light and lean physique. Fast movements, speech, thinking. Excitable, enthusiastic with changing moods. Love excitement and change. Grasp information quickly and forget quickly.	Equally proportioned physique. Forceful nature, low tolerance of disagreement, argumentative, sharp intellect and speech. Likes challenges, enterprising character, efficient.	Heavy and solid physique. Steady energy, do most things slowly and methodically (e.g. eating, digestion etc). Serene, tolerant, forgiving, nature. Slow to grasp information, but retain well.
When under pressure:	Worry, fear and anxiety.	Anger and irritability.	Complacency, inertia, silence.
Seat of imbalances	Colon	Small intestine	Chest
Related body systems and structures	Nervous system and circulatory system. The 'winds' or airs of the body.	Metabolism The heat of the body.	Solid bodily structures and lubrication.
Related health conditions	Anxiety and stress-related conditions, headaches, respiratory conditions, fatigue, tonsillitis, indigestion, wind, colitis, low back pain, high blood pressure.	Heartburn, ulcers, indigestion, jaundice, anaemia, skin inflammation and conditions, heart and circulatory disorders, memory loss, eye diseases and vision problems.	Sluggish digestion, respiratory conditions, low back pain, lethargy, hay fever, sinus problems, joint conditions and laxity.
Things to avoid	Overexertion Anything overexerting that will bring on tiredness and fatigue.	Overeating, strenuous exercise, stimulants (alcohol, caffeine and cigarettes) Anything that adds fuel to the inner fire.	Sweet and cold foods and drinks. Hoarding and holding on to things. Anything that promotes inertia and stagnation.
Work towards:	Sufficient rest, relaxation, quiet time. Regular meals, exercise, meditation, bedtime, water intake. Increase warmth: drinks, baths, showers, light, bright surroundings.	Everything in moderation, eating, exercise, rest, work, leisure. Cool things down: drinks, environments (not too much sunlight), slower pace, time to meditate.	Letting go. Enhance vital energy with regular exercise, healthy eating and manage weight. Try new activities and experiences.

Source: Chopra, D. (1991)

AYURVEDA AND THE DOSHAS

The word Ayurveda originates from Sanskrit language and two root words: *Ayus*, meaning life and *Veda*, meaning knowledge of science. Ayurveda, roughly translates as meaning the 'knowledge or science of life or the life span'. There are many textbooks devoted to the study of Ayurveda. A very brief introduction is provided here.

A key concept in Ayurveda (Indian medicine) is the influence of the mind (see chapter 2), which it is believed can have a powerful influence on health and state of well-being. Ayurvedic practice aims to raise awareness and bring back the connection between mind, body and spirit to create a higher level of health, (Chopra, 1991).

Ayurveda doshas, or the three primary body types, have primary functions and also interconnected functions: vata (controlling movement in the body), pitta (controlling metabolism) and kapha (controlling structures). Table 2.4 lists some of the qualities and characteristics of each type. People may be predominately one type or a combination of two types.

When the doshas are in balance, there is positive health. When there is an imbalance symptoms of poor health develop. The dosha that goes out of balance is often that which is most dominant for the individual.

Stages of disease according to Ayurveda, include:

1. Accumulation: a build up of one or more doshas
2. Aggravation: excess accumulation starts to spread
3. Dissemination: moves through the rest of the body
4. Localisation: settles in an area where it does not belong
5. Manifestation: physical symptoms occur in the area where the dosha has settled
6. Disruption: disease occurs.

Healing takes place through increasing awareness of one's dosha(s), connecting mind, body and spirit, and creating a balanced lifestyle by selecting activities, diet and other lifestyle behaviours that balance one's specific dosha(s).

THE MIND ACCORDING TO YOGA

This section provides an overview of the mind and discusses the effect of kleshas and the ego. Methods used in yoga practice to harness the mind are then discussed, these include: meditation and mantras.

THE MIND (MANAS)

Understanding the concept of the mind has been a source of enquiry for many centuries. The great philosophers (Socrates, Plato, Descartes etc.), psychologists (including Freud, Jung, Beck) and religions (Hinduism, Buddhism etc.) have all contributed to the enquiry.

The mind is the aspect of consciousness that encompasses all mental faculties, which include: thoughts and thinking, perception, reasoning, memory, judgement and imagination. Whether conscious or unconscious, each individual has an inner dialogue or inner voice that processes every life experience, interaction and event, which, in turn, is reflected in their actions, behaviours, beliefs and the way they live and experience their life. Gaining a greater insight and awareness into the processes of one's own mind is a step towards developing a higher level of consciousness. Knowing one's own mind offers the power to restrain some of the processes (e.g. ego and avidya) and impulses (from the senses) that can influence how life is experienced; and enables the making of more positive choices to live a more purposeful life.

The senses

The senses and the sensory organs (eyes, ears etc.) offer the first point of distraction for the mind. We tune in to information from the senses, and the mind and ego can attach all kinds of significances to the information received. The eyes and the ears are those that are most easily distracted by external stimuli. Closing the eyes or focusing on an object withdraws this sense, similarly, chanting a mantra will offer a focus for the sense of hearing until such time that one's inner focus can be maintained and the senses no longer act as a distraction.

The ego (ahamkara)

The ego, or the sense of 'I' is a source of ignorance (avidya). It represents taking all experiences personally and the lower aspect of consciousness. Letting go of ego and attachments is necessary to find the inner and peaceful place.

Intelligence (buddhi)

The higher aspect of consciousness that is able to discriminate and use wisdom to experience and process life and events. It is not attached. It is the wise mind aspect of self, which allows one to be an observer of an experience. It is not enmeshed in the experience. (See mindfulness practice, chapter 9).

For many people, most of the time the mind jumps from one thought to another without any conscious attention or awareness. Each thought creates our reality, how we see and experience life (levels of consciousness or citta). The inner dialogue of the mind has been named the crazy or mad monkey, and the 'chatterbox', (Jeffers, 1998:35) to reflect its endless chattering nature. When the chattering is at full force, we can very easily get swept into a whirlwind experience of different thoughts (who said what, and who did what, this is bad, this is good, etc.) and emotions (fear, anger, excitement, sadness, disappointment, etc.) and connect, usually unconsciously, these thoughts and feelings to memories of similar experiences in the past and our fears and hopes for the future (what if this happens, what about that, etc?). Consequently, all connection to the present moment – the here and now which is always the point and place of power – is lost. Being enmeshed in such thoughts is an act of the ego and blocks the connection to the higher aspect of self, the observer.

The heart and goal of yoga, according to Patanjali, is the 'restraint of all mental modifications', (Sri Swami Satchidananda, 2005:3). That is, gaining awareness of these processes and learning to restrain them, so that they no longer serve to disconnect us from *union* with the higher level of consciousness. Writers and thinkers from different traditions (religion, philosophy, psychology) call this higher consciousness different things: God (Christian and Jewish), Allah (Islam), Shiva, Brahman, Vishnu, Self (Hindu), Buddha nature (Buddhists), Hidden essence (Sufi mystics), universal spirit, soul, higher self, higher mind or higher power (new age spirituality).

> Individuals who are uncomfortable with the term God can use an alternative, e.g. higher power, universe etc. The word God is used because the original source uses the term.

In yoga, meditation (discussed on page 46 of this chapter) is the practice to gain awareness and harness the mind and reach the higher state of consciousness (Raja yoga). A modern-day approach to paying attention is mindfulness (discussed in chapter 9). The exercise in the box opposite offers a simple starting point for getting to know the mind.

THE POWER OF THE MIND

The way we think (our thoughts) will significantly impact the quality of our life experience and the quality of our well-being. Thoughts are energy and they can be used to heal or can create disease (individually and collectively; consciously or unconsciously). Many textbooks are devoted to the connection of the mind and body, the healing process, and collective consciousness. (See the References section in the back of this book for works by: Louise Hay, Caroline Myss, Susan Jeffers, Dan Millman, Deepak Chopra and Wayne Dyer.)

A simple example of the thinking and mind processes is when we are ill or feeling unwell. The most common process is to create thoughts (ego) that reject and resist the pain (e.g. I hate this, I want this to go away etc); these thoughts are often not helpful for the healing process as they focus on those things that are not wanted. If the mind focuses on what it doesn't want, that is what it experiences.

Mindful awareness

Developing an awareness of the mind is the first step towards harnessing a very potent inner power. It is worth taking time to explore and get to know your own mind. Our thoughts affect the quality of our experience and the quality of our life and well-being. This exercise will help you get to know your mind.

- Stop what you are doing, sit comfortably and take a few deep abdominal breaths.
- Spend one minute just taking notice of all the thoughts that pass through your mind. (If you think: 'I am not thinking anything, or this is stupid', then these are thoughts, notice them). Just take the time to notice each thought as it passes through (e.g. I am hungry; I want to get on with reading the rest of this section etc). Notice if you get stuck on a certain thought or if a specific thought keeps popping back into your head. Let go of any judgement about the thoughts and just notice them.
- At the end of the minute, you may want to write down some of the thoughts you remember, just as a way of developing awareness. You can read back over your list of thoughts and consider, if you can think this number of thoughts in one minute imagine how many thoughts you may have over the course of one hour, one day, one week, one month, one year, one lifetime etc!

If you always do what you've always done, you always get what you've always got.

(Source unknown)

For healing, the mind can be used to accept and listen to the messages of the body during illness etc. and can be used to channel more positive thought vibrations by focusing on sending healing, loving and accepting messages that focus on wellness and healing. Doing this shifts the focus of thoughts, which are energy and which impact how we feel and our well-being.

No problem is resolved on the level at which it was created; we must rise to a higher level to find a solution.

(Carl Jung quoted in Myss, 1997:155)

Imagine the body to be like a small child and the mind to be like a parent or best friend. The more you berate, put down or tell a child off 'Don't do this, stop feeling this, etc', the more the child rebels. Whereas, with some attention, acceptance, love and enquiry – wise mind enquiry, *buddhi* ('What is it? What do you need?'), a greater sense of connectedness and the answers to any occasional rebellions (disease) can often be found. However, since many people are quite disconnected from their own body and mind experience, this awareness will take time to develop and demands a patient and nurturing approach (see appendices for healing meditation.)

At present, our Rigpa is like a little baby, stranded in the battlefield of strong arising thoughts. I like to say we have to begin by babysitting our Rigpa, in the secure environment of meditition.

(Sogyal Rinpoche, 1992)

Perception

The mind is subjected to many disturbances (vrittis). These cloud the ability to distinguish between what is transitory (only lasting a short time) and related to the material world, and what is of the spirit (lasting for eternity).

The way we see things or perceive events is always from our own frame of reference and will be influenced by our past experiences, personal history and the society and culture in which we live. We may either believe our perception of a situation is real (ego), when it may not be, or we may ignore our perception of a situation when it is correct and when it would be beneficial to take notice and act. In the Yoga Sutras, this misunderstanding is referred to as 'avidya' (ignorance), meaning that our judgements and actions are clouded. Avidya is believed to be the root cause of all suffering and the root of all other obstacles or kleshas (mental states) that obscure the real self.

The goal of yoga is to still or suppress the thought waves, remove avidya and other obstacles or kleshas, so that we can live to our highest purpose. When this is done through various means suggested in the ancient texts, particularly meditation (discussed later), the self is revealed in its true nature.

That which separates you from God is mind. The wall that stands between you and God is mind. The mind in the vast majority of persons has been allowed to run wild and follow its own sweet will and desire. It is ever changing and wandering. It jumps from one object to another. It is fickle. It wants variety. Monotony brings disgust. It is like a spoiled child who is given too much indulgence by its parents, or a badly trained animal. The minds of many of us are like menageries of wild animals, each pursuing the bent of its own nature and going its own way. Restraint on the mind is a thing unknown to the vast majority of persons.

(Bliss Divine, Swami Sivananda, 1964:288)

KLESHAS

Kleshas are the human impulses and mental states that tend to obscure the self. They are unconscious processes. In Buddhist traditions, they are the roots to all suffering and are blocks to the meditation process. In yoga, it is believed they are the chains that tie the individual into the cycle of rebirth, which prevent the reaching of an enlightened state.

The five kleshas are:

1. **Avidya**: ignorance

Avidya is believed to be the root of all suffering. It is the ignorance of our true nature as spiritual beings, which is often deeply shrouded and hidden and clouded by the other kleshas.

2. **Asmita**: ego

Asmita includes feelings of superiority (top dog), inferiority (underdog) and the way we identify with ourself; which can result in false projections, e.g., 'X is better at this asana than I am'; 'I have to be better at this asana', or 'I know more about this subject then X, I am right, they are wrong' etc. We can become trapped and attached to these projections, rather than just seeing them as a defence of the ego.

3. **Raga**: attachment

Raga is the attachment, attraction to and desire for pleasure and satisfaction, which if not achieved, brings suffering and, if achieved, brings yet another desire or pleasure to fill the gap. For example, we may want things because they felt good the last time we had them (a piece of cake, a relationship, an alcoholic beverage, etc.), even though they may no longer be good for us, and we no longer need these things. Holding on to what we have and not valuing what we have (it is never enough) are examples of raga.

4. **Dvesha**: refusal/rejection

Dvesha is the opposite to raga. It is the aversion, hatred of, rejection and avoidance of anything that causes pain or discomfort. For example, a past experience may have caused a difficulty, so we unconsciously move away from and avoid anything that stirs a similar discomfort (people, places, thoughts, etc.), even though we may have no experience of the new situation. It is staying inside one's comfort zone.

5. **Abhinivesha**: fear

Abhinivesha includes: uncertainty, self-doubt, being afraid that others will judge us, fear of ageing and ultimately, fear of death.

Avidya (and the other kleshas) are not present when we feel peaceful and content, but they are always present when we feel discomfort, unrest and agitation. Awareness, recognition and a friendly acceptance of the kleshas within oneself is the first step towards decreasing their effects and reducing suffering (see Accept, Adjust, Accommodate, chapter 9)

Yoga practice and specifically Kriya yoga (the yoga of action) helps to conquer avidya and help towards purifying the mind to a more enlightened and meditative state. Kriya yoga includes:

1. **Tapas** (cleansing disciplines). Through healthy living and the practice of asanas and pranayama we gain a greater connection with our body – *the physical aspect.*

2. **Svadhyaya** (self-study). Through mindfulness, self-reflection, self-study and study of the scriptures (may include religious texts and more modern self-help books), we gain a greater understanding of ourselves – *the mental aspect.*

3. **Ishvara Pranidhana** (surrender to the divine aspect/quality of action). Through becoming connected to spirit or the divine aspect of self, we live with greater purpose and meaning – *the spiritual aspect.*

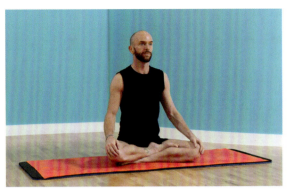

Figure 2.5 Half lotus pose (Ardha Padmasana)

MEDITATION

At a basic level, meditation is quietening of the mind, which enables the meditator to withdraw the senses away from the outer world and focus within, listening to the infinite well of wisdom that lies inside. From this quiet space comes inner peace and a connection to the true self.

Patanjali, (in Fostater & Manuel, 2002:83) describes four meditational states:

- **Pratyahara**: withdrawing the senses (focusing within)
- **Dharana**: concentration (noticing the thoughts and sensations)
- **Dhayana**: meditation (acceptance of all internal experiences and sensations, without having to attach to any; letting go)
- **Samadhi**: absorption. A feeling of great clarity, openness and freedom. The true self (atman).

These states are not linear, nor are they separated by boundaries. During a meditation practice it is possible to move backwards and forwards between states.

> *Meditation is the only royal road to the attainment of freedom. It is a mysterious ladder which reaches from earth to heaven, from error to truth, from darkness to light, from pain to bliss, from restlessness to abiding peace, from ignorance to knowledge, from mortality to immortality.*
>
> Meditation and Mantras,
> Swami Sivananda, 1964:1

BENEFITS OF MEDITATION

Meditation offers a way of finding inner peace and brings many benefits for healing mind, body and spirit.

As discussed earlier, the mind (often the source of discontent and disharmony) offers an endless source of inner chatter, much of which is unconscious. Much like a drunken monkey jumping from tree to tree after being bitten by a spider and stung by a scorpion, the mind flitters from one thought to another.

Every day, the mind is bombarded by stimuli from many directions and through all of our senses (sight, hearing, touch, taste, smell). Advertising force-feeds our ego the illusion of happiness and our desires and wants can grow out of proportion to our actual needs. On top of this the mind is constantly replaying the past, acting out the drama over and over in ever-changing scenarios. Alcohol or drugs are often used to dampen the chatter in a desperate attempt to quiet the mind. Technology has brought us so far and modern lifestyles and privileges are way beyond that of our ancestors, yet inner peace remains an elusive state for many people, most of the time.

Regular meditation brings clarity; it cleanses the mind enabling purer thoughts, motives and intentions. In time, the ego is eradicated, intuition is heightened and hidden knowledge is released from the subconscious bringing wisdom, peace and happiness.

All yogis will admit that meditation is a very high practice. True meditation has profound results that lead to inner quiet, revealed truths and much more. However, meditation can be difficult to practise for many reasons, the main problems include finding it:
- Difficult to sit without pain
- Hard to find focus from the endless, wandering, chatter of the mind
- Too hard not to fall asleep.

Sitting in the traditional seated postures used for meditation can be uncomfortable. Hatha yoga asanas help to train the body and free energy blockages that allow the body to relax and sit more comfortably in meditation. However, this can take a few years. Other traditions use moving meditation (Tai Chi) and mindful movement (e.g. walking meditations, discussed on page 49).

Stilling the chatter of the mind is often the biggest challenge. The mind can be visualised like watching a movie, freeze-framing at certain points, at others rewinding and fast forwarding. Learning to spend time with the thoughts, accepting them, letting them flow, without attaching to a specific thought are ways of working towards creating more stillness. Like throwing a stone in a pond, each thought creates a ripple; we have to learn to reduce the stones and flow with the ripples.

Falling asleep is another barrier to meditation. Rather than sitting with the thoughts and noticing; the level of mental activity created causes exhaustion, so that the minute the eyes close or the body is still, the mind chooses to close down and sleep.

Methods to assist meditation, found by the rishis, include: Samprajnata/Saguna (meaning with seed) and Asamprajnata/Nirguna (meaning without seed) (see Samprajnata/Saguna box over the page).

CONDITIONS FOR MEDITATION

Prior to starting a meditation one should be prepared physically and mentally to turn inwards. Many obstacles that may block regular meditation practice can be removed by following some simple guidelines, which include:
- **Regular time and place**: choosing to meditate at the same time and place daily helps condition and discipline the mind towards the practice. Dusk and dawn are favourable times due to the spiritual energy (see Preferred times for meditation box over the page).
- **Progress steadily**: meditation and stillness is an art. Start with short and regular practices (5–10 minutes) and build gradually to slightly longer durations (20–30 minutes) and eventually to extended durations (1 hour

SAMPRAJNATA/SAGUNA (with seed)

This describes the practice of using a focal point such as a sound/mantra (discussed on page 49) or deity (goddess or god, e.g. Shiva, Buddha, etc.) to help focus the mind and thus allow the thought waves to dissipate. Through constant antar nada (inner sound, e.g. chanting the name of the deity) the mind trains itself, in time, to become eka grata (one pointed or focused). Thoughts and distractions dissolve as the mind becomes trained on one repetition of sound. Often lights are reported as being seen of varying colours around the third eye (ajna chakra) area.

ASAMPRAJNATA/NIRGUNA (without seed)

This describes the practice of meditating by emptying the mind completely (considered a very high practice). This is considered the parama sadhana (highest spiritual practice) and is thought to be achievable by only a tiny minority within the world. In this age of the kali yuga (black age) there are many particles and frequencies distracting our subconscious mind while we remain innocent to its potential detriment.

Preferred times for meditation

Brahma Murhta/Ojas. This is the name given to the spiritual hours between 4 a.m. and 6 a.m. and in the evening time of dusk. These time zones are known to have a more spiritual energy and peace.

Tejas. This means energy and is the energy during the hours of the rest of the day and night.

Renouncing/monk yogis arise at 4 a.m. to help retain the seminal fluid, which in males is secreted naturally around the hours of 4.30 a.m. (known as a wet dream) so as to not release any life force and retain the fluid to build higher spiritual practices.

---

or more). Some individuals may need guided meditations to offer a focus for the mind.
- **No disturbances**: whatever time suits your practice, try to ensure you will not be disturbed. Turn off any mobile phones, lock the doors and make yourself comfortable.
- **Separate space:** try to have a separate area which is only used for meditation as this will allow the positive energy/vibrations to build up there. The area should be regularly cleaned to maintain purity.
- **Create an altar**: an altar can be created by using pictures, statues, symbols, crystals and flowers to create positive energy and focal points. Candles can be burned as light is the purest form of energy. Incense can be burned to create a peaceful atmosphere. Sandalwood oil is often used in temples to purify the mind.

INTRODUCING MEDITATION TO STUDENTS

Meditation can be taught at the beginning or end of any asana practice. Students should have experience of slowing the breath during asana practice before meditation is introduced. In addition:
- The environment should be warm enough to enable everyone to sit comfortably for the length of the meditation. Shawls or warm clothing can be worn if needed.
- The time spent meditating will depend on the

students' experience. For beginners 5 minutes is sufficient and then build gradually over time.
- The position selected must be comfortable to hold for the duration. Beginners or persons with low flexibility or physical limitations can sit in a chair to avoid restlessness and fidgeting.
- Mantras can be used to assist focus.
- Focus points. Objects can be used as points of focus to assist concentration, especially for beginners, e.g. a small statue of your favourite deity, a burning candle, a crystal or picture of the Om symbol.

WALKING MEDITATION

Walking offers an excellent way of achieving a mindful and meditative state, especially in a natural environment (park or rural area, beach or forest) and at quieter times of the day (dawn or dusk). It also offers a good workout for the cardiovascular system.

Silent walking meditations are a regular practice at many ashrams around the world. Each step is taken with a mindful intent, helping to bring peace and quiet to the mind. Mantras can be repeated with each step or over a sequence of steps. Walking meditations are an excellent way to start meditation practice and attain a meditative state, especially for beginners to the practice.

Mantras that can be repeated while walking include:

'**Om Namah Sivaya**', meaning 'Adoration to Siva' repeated over four steps

'**So Ham**', meaning 'I am that, I am' repeated over two steps.

Daily life is not lived in a crossed-legged posture. Eventually we open our eyes and get on with the day. Sitting meditation is a good beginning, enhanced by moving meditation (e.g. Kinhin, Judo, Akido, Tai Chi, walking) which serves as a bridge into everyday life.

Thoughts do not stop arising during moments of dynamic meditation, but we no longer pay homage to them; they lose their power to distract our attention, drive our moods, or weaken our resolve. During dynamic meditation, we liberate our bodies, for the moment, from the mind. Ultimately, everything we do becomes a form of dynamic meditation, and we are freed from the crazy monkey chatter of random thoughts.

Millman, 2006:43

MANTRAS

Mantras are sounds that have a sacred or mystical significance. Mantras may involve single vowel sounds, single words or a series of words, such an affirmation 'all is well' or 'I am peaceful' or a poem or verse, which possess vibrations that allow concentration. Each mantra has a direct effect on the physical body and it is claimed they influence our emotions and mind (removing blocks and obstacles). Some believe that mantras also have an impact on the physical world around us (accumulating abundance, creating peace).

A mantra often relates to a deity without form (Videhas, without bodies) with the mantra being the body. After deep penance the ancient rishis, during meditation, discovered the mantras, which is why the rishis are also known as mantra-darshis (seers of mantras).

Often mantra chanting begins with fingers on one's head where the name of the rishi who discovered the mantra is remembered, then the fingers are placed on the tip of the nose where the name of the mantra is recited and then the fingers are placed on heart where the deity associated with the mantra are remembered, (Ramaswami & Hurwitz, 2006).

Gayatri mantra remembering sequence

Hand placement	Remembering
Fingers on head	Rishi Visamitra
Fingers on nose	Gayatri (the five-faced deity)
Fingers on the heart	Savitur (Brahman as the Sun)

The main purpose of repetition of a mantra is to merge with the deity in absolute concentration, then the qualities of the deity are revealed to the aspirant, (Ramaswami & Hurwitz, 2006).

According to many religious teachings, including Hinduism, the Universe is said to be formed from Divine vibration: 'In the beginning was the word and the word was God', is a well known verse from the Christian scriptures. Every word we speak (as well as every thought we think) resonates through our body and mind, having a positive or negative effect.

Mantras are used to bring about a change in the vibration of the body, mind and spirit. They turn the mind inward toward the divine self and help to release spiritual energy in the chakras. Most commonly, mantras are names of deities (gods and goddesses, e.g. Buddha, Shiva etc), a divine power made manifest. To bring about the desired effects, mantras need to be pronounced correctly and their meaning understood.

Some yoga lineages believe that repeating a mantra all the time will erase bad karma and keep our thoughts towards the divine. Every human cell has a frequency and vibration, mantras are used to harmonise the frequencies and bring balance within and without. They also bring a focal point to yoga practices. Mantras can change consciousness when repeated constantly during meditation, first loudly and then through silent and mental chanting. Internal or silent mantras are thought to be the most powerful.

Different mantra practice includes:
- **Seed mantras or Bijas**. Seed (Bija) mantras are considered the highest practices (as they have no meaning) but have powerful effects due to the vibration of the sound, and are thought to be the sounds of creation itself. These sounds have a subtle effect on our energy channels (nadis) and chakras to help release blockages and awaken the kundalini energy. Once awakened, the energy moves up the spine (sushumna nadi). (Nadis, Chakras and kundalini are discussed earlier in this chapter.) Examples include: Lam, Vam, Ram, Yam, Ham, Ksham, Om to reflect the chakras (see page 35 and chakra meditation in the appendices).
- **Japa** or mantra repetition is used to help focus the mind, free it from the internal chatter and help connect with the Supreme power.
- **Mala beads** (similar to the rosary) are often used to help focus the mind on the mantra. The index finger is not allowed to touch the beads as this is the finger of the ego (the pointing finger). Some yogic traditions believe that to wear your mala beads on display is to boast

to the world you are on a spiritual path. This egotism is considered to be a lack of spiritual understanding and is discouraged. Mala beads should be kept out of sight of others even during japa and for this purpose a special bag can be used to hide the beads from others.
- **Silent mantras** are believed to be the most powerful as they are internalised and therefore personal and private. Saying mantras out loud is equally significant and very powerful when in a group or satsang (spiritual meeting). Please see figure 2.6.

OM AND ITS SIGNIFICANCE

Om is a sacred sound in Hinduism. It is composed of three syllables – A-U-M – which merge into each other. It is a syllable that represents every sound ever uttered and everything that exists: it is the essence of the Universe. The Hindu scripture Mandukya Upanishad is devoted entirely to an exposition of the mysticism of Om.

Om is sometimes called pranava mantra. It is a synonym for the divine principle and is the most powerful of mantras because it represents the first manifestation of the supreme reality or Brahman. The sound is used to preface and end the reading of many sacred scriptures and Hindu prayers and is used in most mantras.

> *AUM is a bow, the arrow is the self, and Brahman (Absolute Reality) is said to be the mark.*
>
> (From: Mandukya Upanishad)

A deeper insight into this mystic symbol reveals that it is composed of three syllables combined into one, not like a physical mixture but more like a chemical combination.

The symbol of AUM consists of three curves (curves 1, 2 and 3), one semicircle (curve 4), and a dot.
- The large lower curve 1 (**Jagrat**), symbolises the waking state and the consciousness is turned outwards through the gates of the senses. The larger size signifies that this is the most common (majority) state of the human consciousness.
- The upper curve 2 (**Sushupti**) denotes the state of deep sleep or the unconscious state. This is a state where the sleeper desires nothing, nor beholds any dream.
- The middle curve 3 (which lies between deep sleep and the waking state) signifies the dream state (**Swapna**). The consciousness in this state is turned inwards, and the dreaming self beholds an enthralling view of the world behind the lids of the eyes.

These three are the states of an individual's consciousness.
- The dot signifies the fourth state of consciousness, known in Sanskrit as **Turiya**. In this state the consciousness looks neither outwards nor inwards, nor the two together. This is the state of absolute quiet, peace and

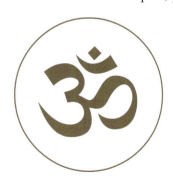

Figure 2.6 OM symbol

bliss, which is the ultimate aim of all spiritual activity. This Absolute state illuminates the other three states.
- The semi-circle separates the dot from the other three curves and symbolises **Maya**. It is the illusion of Maya that prevents us from the realisation of this highest state of bliss. The semi-circle is open at the top, and does not touch the dot, which means that Maya does not affect this highest state. Maya only affects the manifested phenomenon. The effect is that of preventing the seeker from reaching their ultimate goal, the realisation of the One, un-manifest, all-pervading, Absolute principle.

Om chanting

To stimulate the vishuddha chakra (throat chakra)

- Lying (corpse) or seated (sukhasana)
- Close the eyes
- Breathe deeply
- Open the mouth wide and chant 'Aaah' (feel it in the abdomen)
- Round the lips to make the sound 'Ou' (feel the sound move to the chest and throat)
- Close the lips and make the sound 'Mmmm' (feel it in the head and face)

Make each sound last as long as possible Practice initially for 2–5 minutes and progress to 20 minutes.

HATHA YOGA

Hatha yoga originated as a pathway of practice from Raja yoga. In ancient Sanskrit 'Ha' means 'sun' (or left) and 'Tha' means 'moon' (or right). The term 'hatha' is sometimes translated as meaning 'physical' or 'forceful' in that, by performing the asanas and focusing on the breath, the mind is forced to withdraw from external distractions, and instead focuses towards the internal experience, which assists with spiritual awakening.

Hatha (effort) yoga uses the body with varying practices to purify it and attain liberation. Postures, breathing techniques, purification techniques, mantra and meditation are all parts of modern-day Hatha yoga practice, (Satyananda, 1969).

These practices aim at balancing and uniting the energies of the right (pingala) and left (ida) sides and merging them centrally (sushumna) with the spine, prana and apana in the heart centre of the body, (Desikachar, 1999:239) to awaken the kundalini shakti power, a dormant energy situated at the base of the spine, which once awakened, can in turn, awaken the energy centres in the body (chakras) and dormant parts of the brain to expand our consciousness towards our original state. When the kundalini shakti power merges with the shiva energy one attains samadhi (ecstasy/liberation).

The main text used by those who study and practice Hatha yoga is the *Hatha Yoga Pradipika (HYP)*. In Sanskrit, Pradipika means 'light', 'lantern' or 'lamp'. The translated title of the book could be 'An explanation of Hatha Yoga' or 'A light for Hatha Yoga'.

The HYP (as it is commonly known) was originally written around the fifteenth century by an Indian Yogi called Svatmarama – the name 'Svatmarama' means 'one who delights in one's atman'. Little is known about the original author, however, it is believed that he wrote the book by drawing on his own experience and from earlier textbooks (most of which are now lost).

The HYP is an ancient scripture and contains very powerful and unusual techniques to attain liberation. The HYP discusses all the key components of Hatha yoga practice, including: asana or postures; breathing or pranayama; chakras; kundalini; bandhas; kriyas; nadis; mudras and Samadhi. In today's modern life, parts of the HYP are considered dangerous unless one is practising in a sattvic (pure) and spiritual place such as a hermitage. These unusual techniques are often left out of modern-day practice for the safety of the uninitiated or beginner, (Akers, 2002).

Influential gurus

Swami Vishnudevananda

Swami Vishnu-Devananda set up the True World Order and set about training as many people to teach yoga as possible. His philosophy was that the more people taught yoga the more yoga would teach the world how to live with love. Teacher training courses in the Gurukula system (a student lives with their guru/teacher) have been running since the 1970s and over 20,000 yoga teachers have been trained. Training courses are held at ashrams around the world, where the students experience (briefly) the life of renunciation, (Vishnudevananda, 1985).

Swami Vivekananda

Swami Vivekananda is one of the most famous and influential spiritual leaders of the philosophies of Vedanta and Raja yoga and a major figure in the history of Hinduism and India. While he is widely credited with having uplifted his own nation through his teachings, he simultaneously introduced yoga and Vedanta to America and England with his popular lectures and private discourses on Vedanta philosophy. Swami Vivekananda was the first known Hindu Swami to come to the West, where he introduced Eastern thought at the World's Parliament of Religions, in connection with the World's Fair in Chicago, in 1893, (Vivekananda, 1956).

Swami Satyananda Saraswati

Swami Satyananda Saraswati, disciple of Swami Sivananda of Rishikesh and founder of the Bihar School of Yoga, was one of the world's most enlightened yogis of the modern era. He promoted yoga as the 'science of right living', (Satyananda, 1969:1), which worked on all aspects of the individual and when incorporated into day-to-day life benefitted physical, mental, emotional and spiritual health. Today his University of yoga in Bihar, India, still conducts research and evidence of all of yoga's benefits. The light of Yoga shines today because of practitioners such as him and those that went before him.

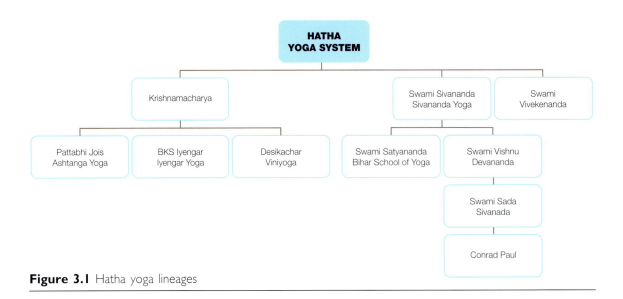

Figure 3.1 Hatha yoga lineages

HATHA YOGA LINEAGES

Yoga (including Hatha yoga) has traditionally been passed on from guru to guru on an individual level. In the beginning it was passed on orally. Then the gurus began to write down their teachings. Eventually, yoga masters began teaching groups of students all aspects of yoga and how to teach it, (Feuerstein, 2003). (See section one, chapter 1: History.)

Today, the well known lineages of Hatha yoga are: Iyengar, Ashtanga vinyasa krama, Viniyoga, Bikram yoga, and Sivananda, all differing in style, (Satyananda, 1969).

Lineages of Hatha Yoga

Sivananda Yoga
Sivananda is a beautiful blend of physical and devotional practices. Each class consists of a little chanting with breathing practices along with asanas of sun salutes and twelve postures. The asana routine is designed to keep the body healthy and the spine strong for more devotional practices and meditation. Today the renouncing order is made up of mainly Western swamis who run the centres and ashrams around the world. The organisation was originally founded by Swami Vishnudevananda who was a disciple of Swami Sivananda Saraswati, who some consider to be a great saint. More emphasis is placed on chanting, breathing and meditation than alignment and props in this style of yoga practice, (Sivananda, 1964).

Viniyoga
The late Sri Tirumalai Krishnamacharya (1888–1989) developed Vinyasa Yoga (linking postures with breathing). A well-known yoga master, Sri Krishnamacharya trained Pattabhi Jois and BKS Iyengar. Over time he developed his approach of gentle linking and flowing of postures. His son TKV Desikachar has carried on his teachings and continued the promotion and proliferation of Vinyasa style yoga, a well-known practice. It is now named the Association of Yoga Studies, (Desikachar, 1995).

Iyengar Yoga
BKS Iyengar has a very precise view of Hatha yoga postures and breathing. In an Iyengar class alignment is everything and pranayama is not introduced until years of asana practice have taken place. As Iyengar believes that the body has its own intelligence, his system works on focusing on physical alignment to help bring balance between mind and body. There may not be much meditation, breath work or chanting in an Iyengar class, as teachers tend to focus on body mechanics rather than on aspects of spirituality, although in BKS Iyengar's books he incorporates all of the Hatha yoga practices, (Iyengar, 2001).

Ashtanga Vinyasa Krama Yoga
Sri K Pattabhi Jois is considered the authority on this style of dynamic Vinyasa Yoga. Nicknamed the 'athlete's yoga' for combining an aerobic workout with strength and dynamism, it combines breath work, asana, drishtis (focal points) and bandhas. Because of this it is not considered a beginner's practice, although one can still start

this practice having no experience whatsoever. As it is a set sequence with the holding of postures it is difficult to adapt the practice with the use of the wall, blocks etc, but it allows for, through repetition of the sequence, the practitioner to dive into the postures without having to think about what to do next, which has enabled home, or self-practice. The 'Primary Series' (the first sequence), consists of 56 Hatha yoga postures linked together using vinyasa (linking postures) and breath work, (Jois, 2010).

Satyananda Yoga

Swami Satyananda Saraswati, a renouncing disciple of Swami Sivananda of Rishikesh, incorporates yoga philosophy and practice to this beautiful style of yoga. The practice combines Hatha yoga in the form of asana, pranayama, cleansing techniques, yoga nidra (yogic sleep practice) and meditative techniques. Founder of the famous Bihar school of yoga, a monastic order dedicated to the science of yoga, Swamiji was a guiding light for many over the last half-century. The Bihar school was the first to introduce a degree in yoga training. Study of the other limbs of yoga is part of this lineage, (Satyananda, 1969).

Bikram Yoga

Bikram Choudhury created 'hot yoga'. The room is usually heated to temperatures of 32–40°C (90–104°F) to help students sweat out toxins and increase the length of their stretches. The routine consists of poses leading into poses, using no props, with few upper body strengtheners and no inversions. Practised in sauna-like conditions, this yoga is not suitable for everyone, especially those with medical conditions, however it is a form of yoga practice that has spread worldwide, (Choudhury, 2007).

PRACTISING ASANA – THE FIRST PART OF HATHA YOGA

Prior to everything, asana is spoken of as the first part of Hatha Yoga. Having done asana one gets steadiness (firmness) of body and mind; diseaselessness and lightness (flexibility) of the limbs.

(*Hatha Yoga Pradipika*)

WHAT IS ASANA?

In Raja yoga, asana (pronounced AAH-sa-na) refers to the sitting position, with the spine straight to allow the correct flow of prana upwards through the Sushumna. In Hatha yoga, asana is 'a specific position that opens the energy channels and psychic centres', (Muktibodhananda, *Hatha Yoga Pradipika*, 1993)

The word asana originates from Sanskrit language and has been translated as meaning 'posture' or 'pose'. These translations are only partially accurate, in that they cannot fully encapsulate the unity of spirit, mindfulness and consciousness that defines asana practice, (Iyengar, 2001). Practice, without the union of breath, body and mind, is arguably not asana.

The Sanskrit word from which asana originates is '*as*', which translated means: 'to be', 'to sit', 'to stay' or 'to be established in a particular position', (Desikachar, 1999:17). Two qualities that need to be present when practising asana, according to Patanjali's Yoga Sutras are:

- **Sthira**: steadiness and alertness in the posture
- **Sukha**: remaining comfortable in the posture.

Without these qualities, there is no asana. For example, a posture that creates physical or mental tension and which cannot be held would not be considered asana; similarly, a posture where the focus of the breath is lost and where the mind and senses are distracted would not be considered asana.

The Yoga Sutras of Patanjali describe '*Sthira sukham asanaṁ*', which translated defines asana as: a posture (Āsanaṁ) which is comfortable (sukham) and steady (sthira), (Satchidananda, 1990:152).

WHY PRACTISE HATHA YOGA AND ASANA?

Hatha yoga (and asana practice) evolved as a way of preparing the body and mind (by developing steadiness and gaining control of the mind) for meditation and maintaining the seated posture. The various postures that have evolved (around

84 in total) have been developed to free the body and unblock any blocked energy (prana).

The spine twisting and bending movements were developed to help individuals regain mobility in the spine; some twisting and bending movements were developed to help release toxins and wind (energy blockages) from inside the body.

Each of the individual postures or asanas offer specific and different holistic benefits and help remove the blockages that prevent the achievement of steadiness and comfort.

In modern life, there are often many physical and mental limitations that prevent a level of comfort and steadiness being achieved. The minute the body is positioned in a certain way, there will be aches, cramps, pains and grumbles experienced.

HOW TO PRACTICE HATHA YOGA AND ASANA

To be considered asana practice, the specific posture being practised should feel comfortable and steady, the breath should flow and the mind should be still (focused on the movement and not distracted with other thoughts). It is therefore essential to start with easier postures that the body and mind feel comfortable with. These can be progressed over time, as strength, flexibility and balance develop. Accepting where one is in the present moment, and our strengths and limitations, is the first step to asana practice.

Asana practice needs to be a mindful practice. The first step of the process is observing and noticing how the body moves without judgement, and with acceptance. This would include:
- noticing where a movement is initiated (which joints? And which muscles?)
- sensing and feeling inefficient movement patterns
- noticing stiffness
- noticing lightness
- noticing the breath
- noticing any blocks to the flow
- noticing any resistance from the mind
- accepting and working with all that is present in the current movement, without judgement.

There are many different postures or asanas; these can be grouped as:
- Standing and balancing postures
- Strengthening and balancing postures
- Side bending (lateral extensions)
- Forward bends (flexions)
- Backward bends (extensions)
- Twisting postures (rotations)
- Inversions (the 'upside down' postures, where the head is lower than the heart)
- Seated postures
- Reclining or lying postures.

THE STRUCTURE OF A HATHA YOGA SESSION

In a Hatha yoga session, all asana practice is structured as:
- preparation for the full pose
- full or main pose
- counterpose.

Preparation pose

These are often an easier or modified version of the full pose and offer a way of preparing the body for the fuller pose. Teaching or practising a preparation pose before the main pose offers a way of layering difficulty and instructions.

Full or main pose

This is the main asana. Concentration and focus needs to be given to moving into the position and working with the breath, holding the position and maintaining the steadiness and breath flow and, finally, moving out of the pose in a way that maintains the flow of steadiness, concentration and grace.

Beginners or individuals who are at that point in time unable to achieve the full pose can repeat the preparation pose as their main pose.

Counterpose (pratikriyasana)

The theme of counterposes, is basically that 'every action has two effects – one positive and one negative', (Desikachar, 1999:27). Counterposes do exactly what they suggest: they counter any possible negative effects of the main asana with the aim being to restore balance and reduce the risk of injury or strain. Counterposes are ideally the simplest possible asana that releases any tension from the main asana.

A guideline for selecting counterposes is to some extent determined by where an individual feels tension after performing an asana; wherever, they feel stiffness, is an indicator that a counterpose may be needed to relieve tension in that specific area. The posture selected will also be determined by the individual's strength and flexibility; beginners will need easier and modified postures.

For some postures, the counterpose may be an opposing movement, for example a counterpose for a strong flexion posture would be a gentle extension posture, and for a powerful back bend, a gentle forward bend. Similarly, a lateral extension or standing balance on the right leg would be a counter movement to a lateral extension or standing balance on the left leg and vice versa.

For some asanas, another asana is the counterpose, e.g., the head stand potentially creates tension in the neck and the lower back (built up from holding the position). The counterposes could be a shoulder stand to release the tension in the neck and child's pose (Balasana) to relieve tension in the lower back.

DRISHTI

Drishti is a focusing technique that assists with looking inwards, towards the self. Directing the gaze at a specific point while practising asanas will assist with concentration and awareness (mindful practice).

Drishti originates from Sanskrit and means sight. The term originates from other Sanskrit words including: drishh – to see, drishau – eye, drishhtim – vision, drishhtah – observed.

In Ashtanga Vinyasa Yoga, there are nine drishti points which are used to offer a point of focus when practising asana. These are:

- The tip of the nose (Nasagrai or nasagram): focus for a standing forward bend
- The navel (Nabi or nabhi Chakra): focus for Downward-facing dog
- The hand (Hastagrai or hastragram): focus for Triangle
- The toes (Padayoragrai or Padayoragram): focus for Seated forward bend
- The thumbs (Angusta ma Dyai or Angushthamadhyam): focus when standing with arms over head
- The sky (Urdhva/Antara Drishti): focus for Warrior 1
- Far right (Parsva Drishti): focus for seated twist to the right

- Far left (Parsva Drishti): focus for seated twist to the left
- The third eye (between the eyebrows – Ajna Chakra/Brumadhya: focus for the tortoise

When practising drishti with asana, the gaze of the eyes should remain soft (i.e., not squinting) to reflect an inner quality of steadiness and stillness. A hard or staring gaze will create tension and hardening and the aim of yoga is to promote softness and release tension and not to intensify any tension. Developing softness creates yielding and promotes connection. Tension and stiffness or hardening, can increase disconnection and a sense of separateness, leading to more stress and anxiety.

Some everyday activities to practise drishti are:
1. Take a moment to direct the gaze and focus on a specific point; this could be a candle flame, a single object in a picture, a leaf on the floor (if outside), a single letter of a word on the page of a book. Be mindful to notice what it is that draws your attention away from focus and makes you look away and direct your gaze elsewhere.
2. Gaze inwardly and focus on the point between the eyebrows (third eye) for one minute.
3. Be mindful and conscious of your gaze and learn to soften and relax the eyes.
4. Observe your wandering eyes, notice what it is that distracts you!

When drishti is practised in synchronicity with the other key components of Ashtanga vinyasa flow (ujjayi breathing and the bandhas, or locks and seals) a state of 'tristana' occurs. Practice becomes graceful yet strong, purifying, flowing and meditative.

BREATHING

Breath control is another important aspect of yoga practice. It is practised at the start and end of the session during initial and ending relaxation (see chapter 7: session structure). It is also practised and should be a focus while performing asanas (see chapter 4 for asana instructions).

The most commonly used breathing techniques when practising asanas are full yogic breath or ujjayi breathing. Pranayama and different approaches to breathing regulation are discussed and explained in chapter 5.

The key for asana practice is that when the breath and posture are united, the mind becomes quieter, enabling an inner focus, which can lead to the development of steadiness and stillness. The external world and all distractions are released and the focus is on the present moment, the here and now.

An awareness of the breath during asana performance can prevent over-exertion and moving too far, too soon. For example, the need to take a quick breath or any loss of the breathing flow or quality may be a sign of over-exertion and an indicator that practice should stop or that a modification is needed.

Nasal breathing, or breathing in and out through the nose, is the most usual practice.
- **Breathing in** when the body and chest are opening, e.g. back bends and lateral extensions, and
- **Breathing out** when the body and chest are closing, e.g. forward flexions and twists.

Developing a steady breathing pattern can be achieved by focusing on the depth and pace of the breath and allowing the breath to become deeper and slower.

Beginners can work with a practice of inhaling for four counts and exhaling for four counts. Intermediate and advanced students can practise more regulated breathing techniques and breath retention, (see Pranayama).

BANDHAS, MUDRAS AND KRIYAS

These are another aspect of Hatha yoga practice and are introduced and discussed in chapter 6. They are locks (bandhas and mudras) or cleansing practices (kriyas).

THE ASANAS OR POSTURES

STANDING AND BALANCING POSTURES

The standing and balancing postures physically energise the body. They help to ground and revitalise the legs and develop strength, poise and balance. The focus on the flow of the breath increases oxygen to the body.

They also help to promote stability and correct posture and alignment. They help to raise awareness of areas where there may be weakness, instability and/or muscle imbalance. The pelvis is the connection between the upper and lower body and in the standing postures, any loss of balance or difficulty getting into or holding a position will indicate where there may be an imbalance, which can then be acknowledged and accepted and developed through practice. Learning to stabilise the pelvis and spine is a step towards mastering the standing and balancing postures.

Psychologically, practising the balancing postures requires concentration and focus. The development of the associated physical skills can help to improve and bring back self-belief and self-confidence. This in turn can help bring back balance to internal and mental systems. When the mind is distracted and off focus, standing balances can be difficult to perform. Regaining the focus offers physical and mental/emotional, or psychological, benefits.

Figure 4.1 Mountain pose or Tadasana
(*Taahd-AAH-sa-ha*, Sanskrit – Tada, mountain)

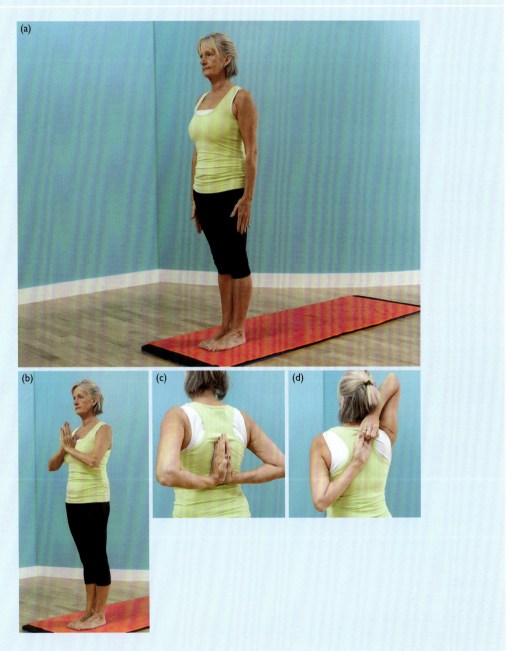

(a) Main posture with hands by sides

Variations:
(b) Hand in prayer position (Samasthiti) – equal standing pose
(c) Hands in prayer position behind back (Tadasana paschima namaskar)
(d) Hands linked behind back in cow position (Tadasna gomukhasana)

Purpose: The foundation and starting position for all other standing postures. Can be used to centre the body before, during and after all standing postures. It is one posture within the sun salutations sequence – Surya Namaskara (sun salutations).

Benefits:
- Improves standing posture, alignment and symmetry
- Improves strength of the legs, thighs and core muscles of the trunk
- Improves balance
- Provides a mental sense of firmness, grounding, stillness and calming

Suitable for: All levels

Precautions:
- Knee hyperextension: keep knees unlocked
- Hip tightness (slightly flexed): encourage full hip extension by engaging buttocks and abductors
- Weak ankles: can use wall or chair for support
- Balance issues: can use wall or chair for support
- Dizziness, low blood pressure: use wall or chair for support and decrease length of time holding position statically

Instructions and teaching points:
- Stand tall with feet together and parallel, big toes touching and heels slightly apart
- Visualise a piece of string attached from crown of head to ceiling and drawing body upwards
- Spread toes and balance weight between both legs equally
- Knees unlocked and thigh muscles draw upwards and rotate slightly outwards
- Pelvis neutral, spine lengthened and abdominals and buttocks engaged
- Shoulder blades slide back and down towards buttocks
- Ears in line with mid-shoulder
- Chin parallel, neck lengthened and crown of head extends upwards
- Breathe softly and deeply

Progressions, modifications and variations:
- Use wall for balance (e.g. Parkinson's, balance issues, vertigo etc.)
- Stand with back against the wall to raise awareness of posture (beginners)
- Wider foot stance (pregnancy, knock knees or foot problems, e.g. bunions
- Seated variation for persons unable to stand, or stand for long durations
- Hand in prayer position (Samasthiti) – equal standing pose
- Hands in prayer position behind back (Tadasana paschima namaskar)
- Hands linked behind back in cow position (Tadasna gomukhasana)

Visualisations:
- Stand firm and tall, visualise roots growing from feet into the earth
- Standing firm as if positioned at the top of a mountain
- Feel the space around the body
- Crown chakra lengthens and opens towards ceiling

Figure 4.2 Upward salute, Raised hand pose or Urdhva Hastasana

(*Oord-vah Hahs-TAH-sa-na*, Sanskrit – Urdhva, raised or upward, Hasta – hand)

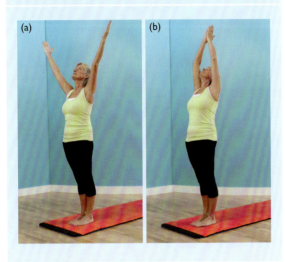

(a) Hands wide above head
(b) Hands in prayer above head

Purpose: A standing and balancing posture. It can be used within preparatory and ending phases. It is one posture within the sun salutation – Surya Namaskara (sun salutations).

Benefits:
- Improves standing posture, alignment and symmetry
- Improves strength of the legs, thighs and core muscles of the trunk
- Improves balance
- Provides mental focus
- Stretches abdominals and pectorals
- Relieves mild anxiety

Suitable for: All levels

Prohibitions: Frozen shoulder

Precautions:
- Shoulder injury: raise hands to smaller range of motion or wide arm position
- Neck injury: look forward
- Knee hyperextension: keep knees unlocked
- Hip tightness (slightly flexed): encourage full hip extension by engaging buttocks and abductors
- Balance issues: can use wall or chair for support
- Dizziness, low blood pressure: look forward rather than upwards

Instructions and teaching points:
- Stand tall in Tadasana
- Inhale
  - Raise arms forwards and upwards into an overhead prayer position
  - Shoulders away from ears
  - Look up and open throat chakra
- Exhale
  - Lower the arms, maintaining prayer position
- Return to Tadasana, arms at side and look forward

Progressions, modifications and variations:
- Stand close to wall or chair if any balance problems
- Look forward, if experiencing dizziness or vertigo
- Widen arms for shoulder discomfort or range of motion issues
- Wider foot stance (pregnancy, knock knees or foot problems, e.g. bunions)
- Seated variation for those unable to stand for long durations, or unable to stand at all
- Lower arm raise, prayer position to forehead or chest, if individual has shoulder range of motion issues

Visualisations:
- Feel the space around the body
- Throat chakra lengthens and opens

Figure 4.3 Tree pose or Vrkshasana

(*Vrik-SHAAH-sa-na*, Sanskrit – Tree or Vrksha)

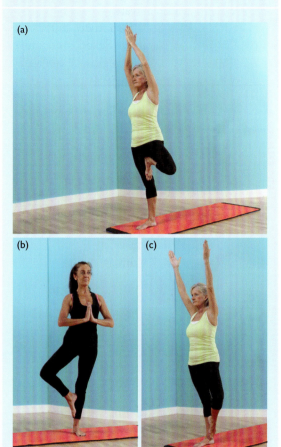

(a) Foot to inner thigh with hands overhead in prayer
(b) Foot to ankle with hand in prayer
(c) Foot to calf with hands wide overhead

Purpose: A standing and balancing posture

Benefits:
- Strengthens quadriceps, gluteals, hamstrings, abductors and gastrocnemius, soleus (supporting leg)
- Strengthens core trunk and spine muscle
- Strengthens deltoids and upper trapezius (arms overhead)
- Stretches adductors and quadriceps (opening hip)
- Strengthens ankles
- Improves flat feet
- Opens the hip area (lifted leg)
- Improves balance
- Improves focus and concentration
- Helps to relive sciatica

Suitable for: All levels, using appropriate modifications

Precautions:
- High blood pressure: keep arms low
- Balance problems: use wall for support
- Knee hyperextension: keep knee unlocked
- Limited hip mobility or rotation: smaller lift and rotation, (i.e. decrease range of motion)
- Pregnancy: keep arms low to avoid raising blood pressure
- Weak ankles: use wall for balance

Instructions and teaching points:
- Stand in Tadasana
- Shift the weight to the right foot
- Support knee unlocked, pull up through the thigh
- Inhale
  - Raise the left foot into the inner thigh, toes point down
  - Extending the spine and ribcage
  - Arms to prayer position at heart centre, chest level
  - Supporting thigh presses against foot
- Exhale
  - Arms raise above head, crown
  - Shoulders away from ears
  - Shoulder blades slide down towards buttocks
  - Chin parallel

- Eyes look forward
- Balance and breathe
- Maintain core engagement

Progressions, modifications and variations:
- Use chair or wall for balance
- Foot position:
  - at side of ankle with toes on floor
  - at side of ankle with toes off floor
  - on calf
  - just above knee
  - tucked into thigh
- Arm position
  - side of body
  - prayer position at chest level
  - single arm overhead: wide
  - double arm overhead: wide
  - both arms overhead in prayer position

Visualisations:
- Stand firm and tall, visualise roots growing from feet into the earth, like a tree
- Hold the position confidently, without judgement
- If your body sways, flow with the movement, like a tree would flow in the wind
- Extend the arms upwards like branches, reaching for the sun
- Crown chakra lengthens and opens towards ceiling
- Imagine the type of tree you would be: a strong oak, a flexible willow

Preparation: Modified or easier variation

Counterpose: Opposite side

Figure 4.4 Warrior 2 or Virabhadrasana 2

(*Veera-bhad-rah-sa-na*, Sanskrit – Virabhadra, a mythological warrior or sage)

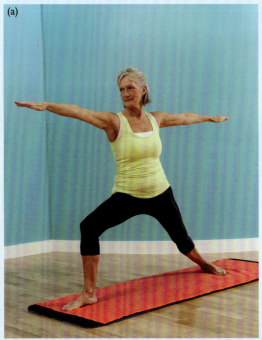

(a)

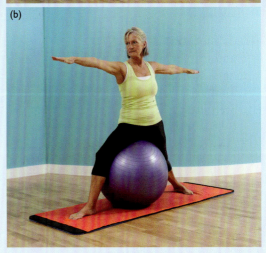

(b)

(a) Full posture

Variation:

(b) Using chair or ball

Purpose: A standing balancing and strengthening posture

Benefits:
- Strengthens the quadriceps, gluteals and hamstrings on supporting leg
- Strengthens ankles
- Strengthens trunk and core muscles of the abdominals and spine
- Strengthens deltoids and upper trapezius (arms lifted)
- Stretches the adductors, gastrocnemius and hip flexor
- Improves balance and concentration
- Provides focus and grounding

Suitable for: All levels

Precautions:
- Knee problems: smaller knee bend
- Neck: look forward without rotation
- Shoulders: hands on hips
- High blood pressure: hands on hips or in prayer

Instructions and teaching points:
- Stand in Tadasana
- Inhale
  - Turn left
  - Step the left foot wide to the end of the mat
  - Left foot at a 90° angle
- Exhale
  - Rotate left thigh outward
  - Right foot faces forward
  - Chest and hips face left
  - Spine long
- Inhale
  - Raise arms to shoulder height
  - Shoulders away from ears
  - Neck lengthened
- Exhale
  - Bend left knee
  - Left thigh parallel to floor (or as close as possible)
  - Push energy though both legs
  - Look to the middle finger of left hand (drushti)
  - Neck and spine long
  - Chin parallel to the floor
- Hold position and breathe naturally

Progressions, modifications and variations:
- Narrower stance
- Smaller knee bend
- Hands on hips
- Sit on a chair or ball to support body weight
- Progress to half moon pose

Visualisations:
- Visualise having the strength of a warrior in the pose
- Keep the feet strongly grounded and the body firm and flexible
- Look to index finger of front hand (Drushti)
- Maintain a strong focus

Preparation: Modified version

Counterpose: Same posture on opposite side

Figure 4.5 Warrior 1 or Virabhadrasana 1
(*Veera-bhad-rah-sa-na*, Sanskrit – Virabhadra, a mythological warrior or sage)

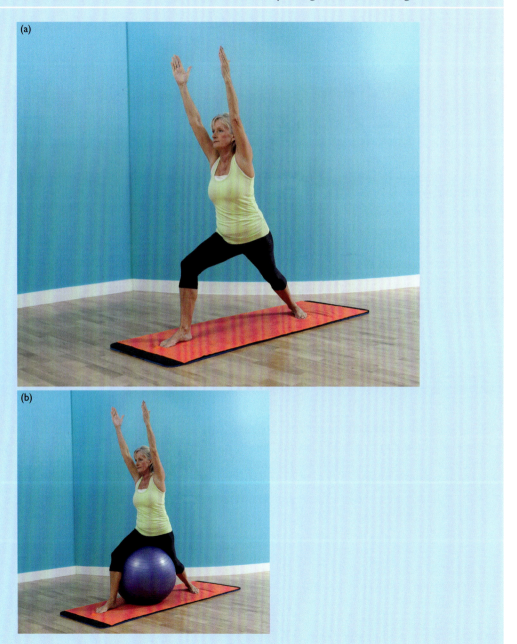

(a) Full posture

Variation:

(b) Using chair or ball

Purpose: A standing balancing and strengthening posture

Benefits:
- Strengthens the quadriceps, gluteals, hamstrings
- Strengthens the ankles
- Strengthens the core and trunk muscles
- Strengthens deltoids and upper trapezius (arms raised)
- Stretches the gastrocnemius, soleus, adductors, hip flexor and latissimus dorsi
- Improves balance and concentration
- Opens the anterior (front) of the body

Suitable for: More advanced. This is an advanced version of Warrior 2

Precautions:
- Knee problems: smaller knee bend
- Back: avoid arching back and place hands on hips
- Neck: look forward
- Shoulders: hands on hips
- High blood pressure: hands on hips or in prayer

Instructions and teaching points:
- Stand in Tadasana
- Step the left leg back about three feet, keep both legs straight, with knees unlocked
- Turn left (back) foot to 90° angle (for a beginner) or 45° angle (more advanced)
- Hips face forward
- Inhale
  - Raise arms above head with palms together
  - Shoulders back and down away from ears
  - Space between ribcage and pelvis
  - Abdominals engaged
- Exhale
  - Bend the right (front knee) in line with ankle and sink downwards
  - Weight balanced through both feet and legs
  - Look upwards (opening throat chakra) without dropping head back
  - Keep arms visible
- Breathe comfortably

Progressions, modifications and variations:
- Narrower stance
- Smaller knee bend
- Hands on hips
- Hands at chest level in prayer
- Perform using stability ball or chair
- Progress to Warrior 3

Visualisations:
- Visualise having the strength of a warrior in the pose
- Keep the feet strongly grounded and the body firm and flexible
- Look to index finger of front hand (Drushti)
- Maintain a strong focus

Preparation: Modified version

Counterpose: Opposite leg

Figure 4.6 Warrior 3 or Virabhadrasana 3
(*Veera-bhad-rah-sa-na*, Sanskrit – Virabhadra, a mythological warrior or sage)

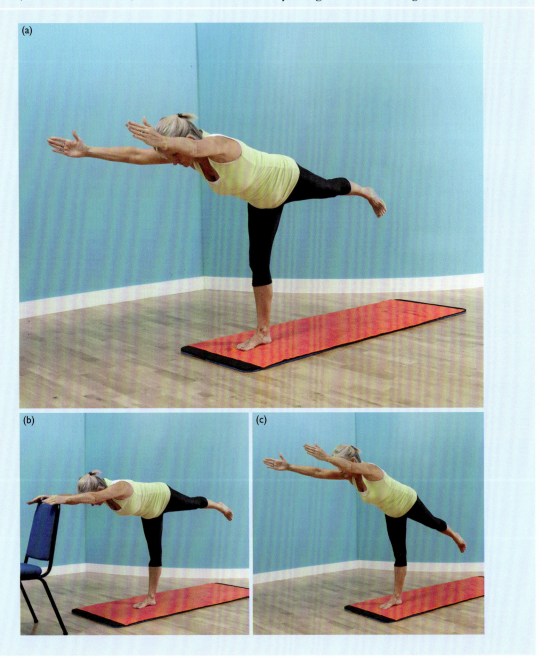

(a) Full position
(b) Modification – holding chair or wall
(c) Modification – smaller lift

Purpose: An advanced standing, balancing and strengthening posture

Benefits:
- Strengthens the quadriceps, gluteals, abductors
- Strengthens the ankles
- Strengthens trunk and core muscles
- Strengthens posterior deltoids, upper and middle trapezius (arms extended)
- Stretches the calf, hamstring, inner thigh, hip flexor and latissimus dorsi, pectorals
- Improves balance and concentration
- Grounding

Suitable for: Advanced

Prohibitions:
- Those experiencing vertigo, dizziness, balance problems, high blood pressure, lower back pain

Precautions:
- Back: smaller forward lean, keep foot on floor, avoid arching back and place hands on hips
- Shoulders: hands on hips
- High blood pressure: hands on hips or in prayer
- Balance: to assist balance can use chair or ballet barre

Instructions and teaching points:
- From Tadasana, step into Warrior 1 position
- Inhale
  - Raise arms above head with palms together
  - Shoulders back and down away from ears
  - Raise the back heel keeping toes on the floor
- Exhale
  - Bend forward from hips, lengthening forward
  - Chest as close to thighs as possible, so body is parallel to floor
  - Arms lengthened and neck in line
  - Eyes look to floor
  - Shift weight to front leg, keeping back toes on floor for balance
- Inhale
- Raise back leg parallel to floor
- Hips square and facing floor
- Extend front knee (knee unlocked)
- Lengthen crown of head away from heel
- Breathe naturally

Progressions, modifications and variations:
- Start with Warrior 1 pose
- Lift leg slightly away from floor initially
- Hands on hips
- Use wall, chair or ballet barre for balance (both hands holding initially and then one hand)
- Hands supported on thighs or hands out to side of body (aeroplane)
- Smaller forward bend

Visualisations:
- Visualise having the strength of a warrior in the pose
- Keep the feet strongly grounded and the body firm and flexible
- Look to index finger of front hand (Drushti)
- Maintain a strong focus

Preparation: Warrior 1 or any modification

Counterpose: Opposite leg

Figure 4.7 Garland pose, Hindi squat pose, Frog pose or Malasana

(*Mal-AAH-sa-na*, Sanskrit – Mala: bead or garland)

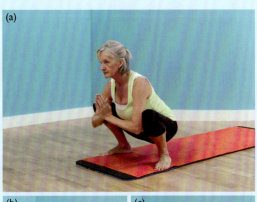

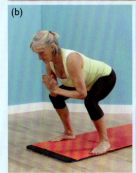
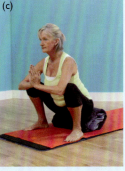

(a) Full position
(b) Modification – knees at 90 degrees
(c) Modification – seated on blocks

Purpose: To mobilise and open up the hips and knees

Benefits:
- Stretches adductors, gluteals and groin area, soleus and lower calf area (when in squat position)
- Strengthens quadriceps and gluteals (lowering into position)
- Strengthens core to maintain posture
- Opens pelvic area
- Massages internal organs

Suitable for: All levels

Prohibitions:
- Knee injury and arthritis
- Hip replacement
- Achilles injuries

Precautions:
- Knee problems: smaller bend, 90° angle at knee
- Tight calves: raise feet on blocks or towel under feet

Instructions and teaching points:
- Stand in Tadasana
- Widen feet and slight turn out of toes (10 to 2 on clock face)
- Place hands in prayer position at chest level
- Inhale and lower buttocks to the floor
- Spine stays long and crown of head towards ceiling
- Elbows inside knees to open hips
- Exhale
- Relax into position
- Breathe comfortably and hold position
- Exhale to return to standing position

Progressions, modifications and variations:
- Use supine lying variation as non-weight bearing option for hip or knee problems
- Squat to a 90° angle to reduce weight bearing on knees
- Squat to sit on blocks to assist weight bearing

Visualisations:
- Feet strongly grounded to the floor
- Feel the spine lengthen and the hips open

Preparation: Mountain pose

Counterpose: Mountain pose

Figure 4.8 Chair pose, Fierce pose or Utkatasana

(*Oot-khut-AAH-sa-na*, Sanskrit – Utkata: fierce, powerful)

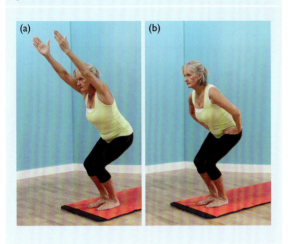

(a) Full with arms extended and deeper bend

Variation:
(b) With hands on hips or single arm raise

Purpose: A standing, strength and balance posture

Benefits:
- Strengthens quadriceps, hamstrings, gluteals, erector spinae, abdominals, deltoids, upper and lower arm
- Lengthens latissimus dorsi and obliques
- Mobility for shoulders, hip and knees
- Increase body temperature
- Stimulates the diaphragm and heart
- Improves flat feet and strengthens ankles

Suitable for: All levels

Precautions:
- Knee problems: take a smaller bend
- Limited ankle mobility: smaller bend and use block under heels
- Lower back pain or hip pain: take a smaller bend
- Shoulder problems: keep arms by side of body or in prayer position at chest level
- Low strength: shorter hold and perform as flowing sequence with Tadasana, smaller bend, can perform with chair, hands on thighs

Instructions and teaching points:
- Stand in Tadasana and ground feet
- Inhale and place hands on thighs
- Exhale and slide hands down thighs and bend at knees and hips into a seated-on-chair position
  - Knees and ankles together
  - Knees in line with toes, without over shooting
  - Hands rest just above the knees
  - Chest forward to the hips, creating a 'Z' or thunderbolt shape
- Inhale
  - Raise arms upwards in line with spine and in a prayer position
  - Keep abdominals engaged
  - Look towards the thumbs to open the throat chakra
- Neck long, throat and face relaxed
- Exhale
- Breathe comfortably to hold position

Progressions, modifications and variations:
- Smaller bend
- Hands on thighs or in prayer
- Arms over head wide or in prayer
- Look forward or upwards

Visualisations:
- Feet firm and grounded
- Feel strong through the thighs
- Lengthen through the spine
- Arms lengthened and extended

Preparation: Smaller bend and range of motion

Counterpose: Mountain pose (Tadasana), Forward bend (Uttanasana)

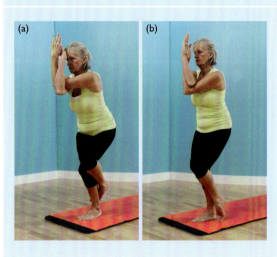

Figure 4.9 Eagle pose or Garudasana
(*Ga-rood-AAH-sa-na*, Sanskrit – Garuda, eagle)

(a) Full position
(b) Modification – wrap of arms and legs without knee bend

Purpose: A standing and balancing posture.

Benefits:
- Strengthens the quadriceps, gluteals, hamstring, gastrocnemius, soleus, erector spine and abdominals
- Stretches abductors, tibialis anterior, posterior deltoid, and trapezius, rhomboids
- Improves balance and concentration
- Stimulates lymph and circulatory systems

Suitable for: More advanced

Prohibitions:
- Hip and knee replacement or injuries
- Shoulder injuries
- Limited balance

Precautions:
- Ankle problems: perform without ankle wrap
- Balance problems: use wall or chair for balance

Instructions and teaching points:
- Stand in Tadasana with feet grounded and connected
- Exhale
  - Bend at knees and hips into a chair seated position
  - Engaging abdominals
- Inhale
  - Transfer weight to the right leg
  - Lift left leg and cross over the thigh, wrapping ankle under the right calf, if possible
- Exhale
  - Extend from hips
  - Lengthen spine and engage abdominals
  - Chin tucked in
- Inhale
  - Raise arms to shoulder height and bend elbows to a 90° angle
  - Draw the elbows in together
  - Bring the left arm under the right arm and rotate the left palm and right palm together
  - Keep elbows in line with shoulders
- Breathe comfortably to hold and relax into the position

Progressions, modifications and variations:
- Isolate and perform arm position in Tadasana
- Wrap legs and arms without bending balancing leg
- Isolate leg position and place hands on thighs
- Use wall or chair for balance

Preparation: Modified positions and isolation of legs and arms before main pose

Counterpose: Opposite side

Figure 4.10 Extended hand to big toe pose or Uttihita Hasta Padangusthasana

(*Oo-TEET-uh Haws-tuh Pod-ung-goos-TAW-sa-na*, Sanskrit – Uttihita, extended; Hasta, hand; Padangusthasana, big toe)

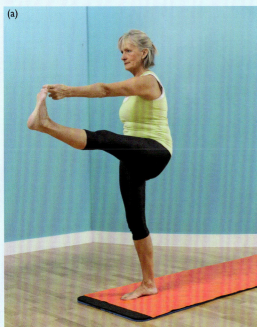

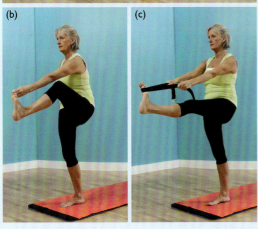

(a) Full position
(b) Modified version – bent knee and leg closer
(c) Modification using strap to support foot

Purpose: A standing and balancing posture

Benefits:
- Strengthens quadriceps, gluteals, hamstrings and gastrocnemius (supporting leg)
- Stretches hamstrings and gluteals (on the held, extended leg)
- Strengthens core abdominal muscles and erector spinae to hold position
- Improves balance
- Strengthens ankles

Suitable for: Advanced

Prohibitions: Not recommended for individuals with limited flexibility in hamstrings or balance problems, or persons with sciatica

Precautions:
- Balance issues: use wall or chair for support
- Flexibility limitations: bend stretching leg and use modifications

Instructions and teaching points:
- From Tadasana
- Shift the weight to the right leg and balance by firmly rooting foot to the floor
- Hips face forward and pull up through the supporting thigh
- Keep spine long
- Right hand on hip
- Bend left knee and grasp left big toe with two fingers (forefinger and middle finger) curling around toe
- On an exhale extend the leg
- Keep the spine long and look forward
- Dorsi-flexing the foot
- Breathe comfortably to hold balance
- Lower on an inhale

Progressions, modifications and variations:
- Use wall or chair to assist balance
- Knee bent on stretching leg to reduce range of motion
- Bend supporting knee to assist balance and stretch
- Use a strap around foot
- Progression: take the leg to the side to open up the hip (stretching adductors)

Visualisations:
- Bring the leg to a right angle with the floor
- The arm that reaches for the toe creates a strong triangle shape with the chest and thigh

Preparation: Smaller range of motion

Counterpose: Mountain pose (Tadasana), Forward bend (Uttanasana)

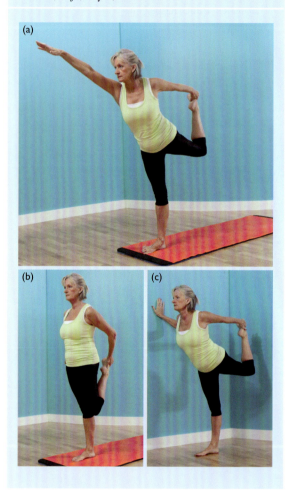

Figure 4.11 Dancer's pose, King of the dance pose or Natarajasana
(*Nat-ahh-raaj-AHH-sa-na*, Sanskrit – Nata, dancer; raja, royal)

(a) Full position
(b) Modification – quad stretch
(c) Modification – using wall for balance

Purpose: A standing balancing, back-bending posture that offers strengthening and flexibility

Benefits:
- Strengthens quadriceps, gluteals, hamstrings, gastrocnemius, soleus, shoulder and upper back (supporting leg and lifting arm)
- Strengthens erector spinae and core stabilisers
- Stretches quadriceps, hip flexor, abdominals, pectorals, shoulder, (stretching side)
- Improves balance and concentration
- Opens chest – heart chakra
- Back bend
- Provides grounding

Suitable for: More advanced. Beginners can use modified positions

Prohibitions:
- Lower back problems, use modifications

Precautions:
- Lower back pain: limit spine hyperextension
- Knee hyperextension: keep knee unlocked
- Balance problems or flat feet: use wall or chair to assist balance

Instructions and teaching points:
- Stand in Tadasana
- Inhale
  - Shift weight onto right leg and raise left leg to buttocks, take hold of ankle (quadriceps stretch)
  - Support knee unlocked
- Exhale
  - Bend the right knee and gently arch the back into a bow shape
  - Take the heel away from the buttocks
- Inhale
  - Raise the right arm upwards, palm faces in towards body
- Exhale
  - Lengthen the body forwards
  - Extending arm and stretching leg should move away from each other
- Keep space between the vertebrae
- Breathe comfortably and hold position

Progressions, modifications and variations:
- Basic quadriceps stretch
- Use wall for balance
- Use a strap or band around lower leg

Visualisations:
- Balancing leg is strongly grounded and rooted to the earth
- Open the body with grace
- Focus gaze forward

Preparation: Single leg quadriceps stretch

Counterpose: Forward bend (Uttanasana)

TWISTING POSTURES

The twisting and rotating postures provide mobility for the spine and can help to alleviate some of the effects of slouching by stretching the muscles around the spine and focusing on correct posture. Maintaining spine mobility also assists with promoting deeper and fuller breathing, using more of the lungs.

The rotating postures also target the internal organs and work deep inside the body, massaging and twisting the organs, to literally wring out any blockages, remove toxins and promote cleansing. They encourage increased blood flow when the posture (or twist) is opened and realigned, providing a refreshing release. This in turn can help to increase levels of energy.

Psychologically, emotional and mental tensions that contribute to 'feeling blocked' can also be released. Strong emotions, such as fear or anger, can be squeezed and visualised as being 'let go', which can lead to freedom and courage.

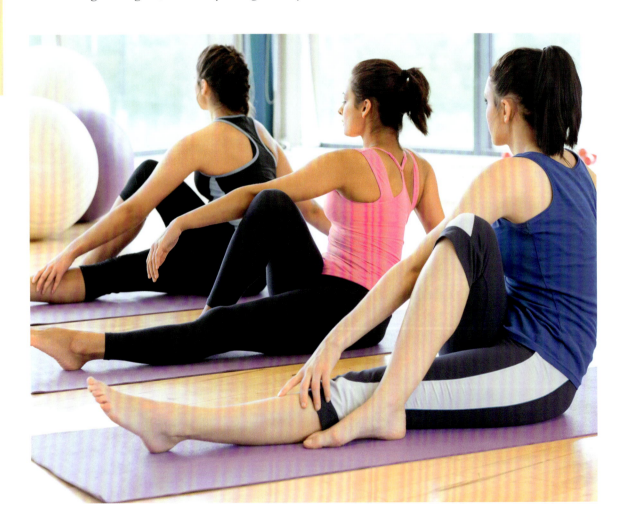

Figure 4.12 Twisting chair pose or Parivrtta Utkatasana

(*Par-ee-vrt-tah Oot-kah-tah-TAHH-sa-na*, Sanskrit – Parivrtta, twist; Utkatasana, chair pose)

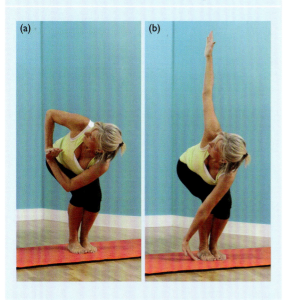

(a) Full position with hands in prayer
(b) Full position with hands in crucifix

Purpose: A standing balancing, strengthening and twisting posture

Benefits:
- Strengthens quadriceps, hamstrings, gluteals, erector spinae, abdominals, deltoids, upper and lower arm
- Stretches obliques on rotation
- Mobility for shoulders, hip, spine and knees
- Increase body temperature
- Stimulates digestion
- Improves flat feet and strengthens ankles

Suitable for: Intermediate

Precautions:
- Knee problems: take a smaller bend
- Limited ankle mobility: smaller bend and use block under heels
- Lower back pain or hip pain: take a smaller bend and avoid rotation
- Shoulder problems: keep arms by side of body or in prayer position at chest level
- Low strength: shorter hold and perform as flowing sequence with Tadasana, smaller bend, can perform with chair, hands on thigh

Instructions and teaching points:
- Stand in Tadasana and make sure feet are grounded
- Move into chair pose
- Inhale
  - Squeeze thighs together
  - Hands in prayer position
- Exhale
  - Rotate one elbow to outside of opposite knee
- Breathe comfortably and hold position
- Twist can be increased on exhale
- From Tadasana repeat on other side

Progressions, modifications and variations:
- Chair pose without twisting
- See chair variations
- Arms can open in crucifix position in twisted position to increase obliques stretch and bring in a pectoralis stretch

Visualisations:
- Feet firmly grounded
- Lengthening through spine
- Rotation, wrings out tension and energy blocks

Preparation: Chair

Counterpose: Opposite side or forward bend (Uttanasana)

Figure 4.13 Triangle pose or Uttihita Trikonasana

(*Tree-khon-AAH-sa-na*, Sanskrit – Utthit, extended; Tri, three; Kona, angle)

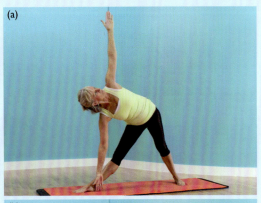

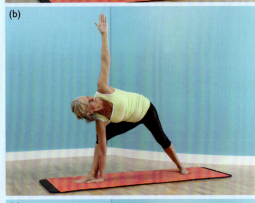

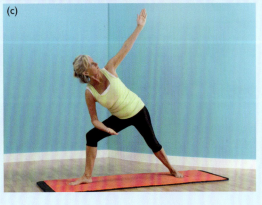

(a) Full position
(b) Modification – Bent knee and arm lifted with hand on floor
(c) Modification – Bent knee with elbow on knee and arm lifted

Purpose: Standing posture with lateral extension and rotation

Benefits:
- Strengthens quadriceps, gluteals, and lower legs (holding position)
- Strengthens trunk and core to maintain spine alignment
- Increases mobility in the hips, spine, shoulder and neck
- Lengthens and stretches hamstrings, obliques and pectorals in full triangle position
- Trunk rotation massages internal organs (abdominal and colon region)
- Stimulates digestion
- Relives menopausal symptoms

Suitable for: All levels. Beginners should start with modified position

Prohibitions: Diarrhoea, high or low blood pressure, neck problems, headaches, pregnancy

Precautions:
- Lower back mobility problems: use modified position with bent knee and limit range of motion
- Shoulder pain: keep arm at side or place hand on hip
- Neck mobility issues: look forward
- Vertigo or dizziness: look forward (and possibly smaller range of motion)
- Knee hyperextension: keep knees unlocked
- Limited flexibility: use blocks or chair for hand or modified position

Instructions and teaching points:
- Stand in Tadasana
- Step the feet shoulder width and a half apart
- Hips face forward
- Spine lengthened
- Right foot turns to 90° angle
- Left foot turns slightly inwards, heel rotates away from right foot
- Knees unlocked
- Chest and hips face left
- Inhale
  - Raise arms to shoulder height
  - Shoulders away from ears
  - Neck lengthened
- Exhale
  - Extend torso to right, bending out of hips
  - Right arm reaches down right leg, as far as comfortable (right hand can be placed on floor behind calf or right index finger can wrap around the right big toe with thumb at the top of big toe)
- Inhale
  - Left arm raises to ceiling, in line with right arm
  - Open chest
  - Palm faces forward
- Exhale
  - Rotate shoulder back and down and open chest and hips
  - Look upwards towards middle finger of left hand
- Breathe comfortably and hold

Progressions, modifications and variations:
- Use modified bent knee position initially
- Hand on thigh, rather than elbow (in modified position to decrease range of motion)
- Look forward if having balance issues
- Shoulder problems – keep arms down and visualise lengthening through arm and side
- Progress to straight leg with hand on leg initially
- Progress to hand on floor and index finger wrapping around toe
- Can place hand on blocks or chair to decrease range of motion

Modification instructions:
- Exhale
  - Bend right knee, thigh parallel to floor (as close to as possible)
  - Push energy though both legs
  - Lower right elbow to right knee (can use forearm to prevent knee from rolling in)
- Inhale
  - Left arm raises to ceiling, in line with right arm
  - Open chest
  - Palm faces forward
- Exhale
  - Rotate shoulder back and down and open chest and hips
  - Look upwards towards middle finger of left hand
- Breathe comfortably and hold

Visualisations: Focus gaze towards middle finger or extended arm

Preparation: Warrior 2 or any of the modifications of triangle listed

Counterpose: Same posture on opposite side

Figure 4.14 Revolved triangle pose or Parivrtta Trikonasana
(*Par-ee-VRT-ta Tree-khon-AAH-sa-na*, Sanskrit – Parivrtta, other side, turn around, revolve; Utthit, extended; Tri, three; Kona, angle)

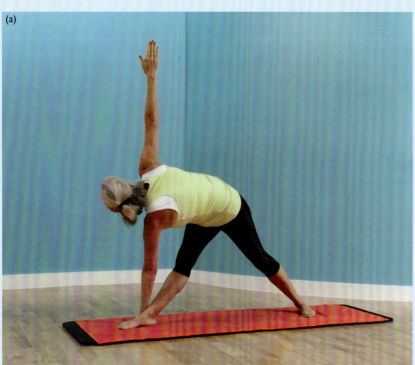

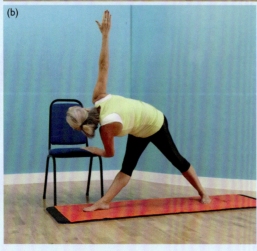

(a) Full position

(b) Revolved triangle with hands on chair to support balance

Purpose: Standing posture with lateral extension and rotation

Benefits:
- Strengthens quadriceps, gluteals, and lower legs (holding position)
- Strengthens trunk and core to maintain spine alignment
- Increases mobility in the hips, spine, shoulder and neck
- Lengthens and stretches hamstrings, erector spinae, obliques and pectorals in full position
- Trunk rotation massages internal organs (abdominal and colon region)
- Stimulates digestion
- Relieves menopausal symptoms

Suitable for: Advanced

Prohibitions: Diarrhoea, high or low blood pressure, neck problems, headaches, pregnancy, prolapsed disc, vertigo or dizziness, sciatica

Precautions:
- Lower back mobility problems – use blocks or chair for hand or modified position
- Knee hyperextension – keep knees unlocked
- Limited flexibility – use blocks or chair for hand or modified position

Instructions and teaching points:
- Stand in Tadasana
- Step the feet shoulder width and a half apart
- Hips face forward
- Spine lengthened
- Right foot turns to a 90° angle
- Left foot turns slightly inwards, heel rotates away from right foot
- Knees unlocked
- Chest and hips face left
- Inhale
  - Raise arms to shoulder height
  - Shoulders away from ears
  - Neck lengthened
- Exhale
  - Extend torso to right, bending out of hips
  - Bend right knee
  - Left hand to floor by the side of the right foot
- Inhale
  - Right arm raises to ceiling to face back of room, rotating from spine
  - Open chest
- Exhale
  - Straighten the front leg (option to keep bent)
  - Look upwards towards middle finger of left hand
- Breathe comfortably to hold position

Progressions, modifications and variations:
- Start in Warrior 2 pose
- Move into Triangle pose
- Bend knee, rather than keeping leg straight
- Use a block to support balance
- Hand on a chair to support balance

Visualisations:
- Focus gaze towards middle finger or extended arm (Drushti)

Preparation: Triangle

Counterpose: Opposite side

Figure 4.15 Half lord of the fishes pose or Ardha Matsyendrasana

(*ARD-Ha Matsy-en-DRAAH-sa-na*, Sanskrit – Ardha, half; Matsy, fish; Endra, ruler, lord)

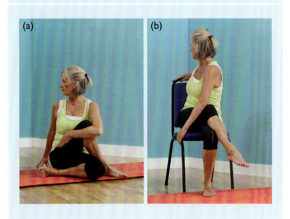

(a) Full position
(b) Modification – chair seated version

Purpose: A seated, twisting posture

Benefits:
- Stretches obliques and abductors
- Opens chest and shoulders
- Mobilises spine and hip and knees
- Improves seated posture
- Strengthens abdominals and core muscles
- Massages internal organs
- Rotations wring out tension from body

Suitable for: Intermediate

Prohibitions:
- Pregnancy
- Hernia

Precautions:
- Lower back problems: can twist away from bent leg
- Knee problems: lower leg extended
- Neck problems: look forward
- Hip problems: use sukhasana and sit on a block

Instructions and teaching points:
- From hero (see page 125) with hands each side of buttocks
- Lift buttocks over to the right side onto floor
- Lift left leg over right thigh, foot flat on floor by knee
- Left buttock to floor
- Left hand on floor close to buttocks
- Inhale
  - Extend right arm up
- Exhale
  - Rotate left shoulder and face left hand side of room
  - Right arm extends outside of right knee
  - Rotate a little further
  - Shoulders square
- Eyes closed in final position
- Breathe comfortably to hold position

Progressions, modifications and variations:
- Keep lower leg straight (Marichyasana or Marichi's pose or Sage's pose)
- Use hands to bring knee to chest and small rotation
- Twist away from bent leg
- Rotate in sukhasana, cross-legged position
- Sit on a chair and rotate or twist spine
- Standing rotations/twists

Visualisations:
- Maintain length through the whole spine
- Imagine any tension, stress or anger being squeezed out
- Open the chest and heart chakra
- Crown chakra extends upwards
- Release any knots and blockages

Preparation: Smaller range of motion

Counterpose: Opposite side

LATERALLY EXTENDING POSTURES

The side bending and lateral postures share many of the effects and benefits of the standing postures. However, they also demand great levels of flexibility to get into the positions and great levels of strength and endurance to hold the positions. They are often more demanding on the cardiovascular system, as the length of the levers (extra weight) being moved and held will demand greater levels of oxygen to be supplied and the heart will need to work harder to accommodate this demand.

Psychologically, these postures require great concentration and awareness of how the physical body moves. Developing the skills to perform these postures can increase confidence and a sense of mastery.

Figure 4.16 Extended side stretch or Utthita Parsvakonasaana

(*Oot-t-hee-tuh Paarsh-ovak-kohn-AAH-sa-na*, Sanskrit – Utthita, extended; Parshva, side)

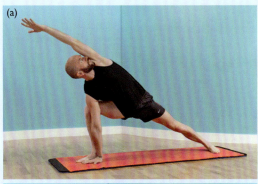

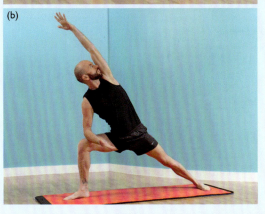

(a) Full position
(b) Modification – elbow on knee

Purpose: Standing lateral bending posture

Benefits:
- Stretches adductors, obliques, latissimus dorsi, hip flexor (stretching side)
- Strengthens quadriceps and gluteals (supporting bent leg)
- Strengthens core muscles of abdominals and spine to maintain posture
- Strengthens deltoid and upper trapezius (lifted arm)
- Opens up chest, hip, groin and side of body
- Massages internal organs
- Improves balance

Suitable for: More advanced (full posture); other levels use modified position

Prohibitions:
- Balance problems: use modified position
- Pregnancy: use modified position

Precautions:
- Neck strain or dizziness: look forward rather than upwards
- Knee injuries: smaller bend
- Hip tightness: use modified position or Warrior 2

- Low flexibility: use modified position or Warrior 2

Instructions and teaching points:
- From Warrior 2
- Exhale
  - Bend to one side extending from the hips
  - Elbow on thigh, shoulders square and away from ears
- Inhale
  - Extend arm overhead, keeping a straight line from finger tip to ankle
  - Look upwards towards armpit
  - Spread weight equally, push energy through back heel
- Exhale (progression)
  - Place hand on floor, outside of the foot
  - Lower body to create a ski slope from finger to toes
- Breathe comfortably

Progressions, modifications and variations:
- Warrior 2
- Smaller knee bend
- Hand on thigh and side bend
- Elbow on thigh and side bend
- Seated on stability ball or chair

Visualisations:
- Create a straight line from little finger to toe on the extended side
- Visualise the line of the body as a ski slope

Preparation: Warrior 2 or any modification listed

Counterpose: Same posture on opposite side

Figure 4.17 Half moon pose or Ardha Chandrasana

(*Ar-dhuh Chan-DRAAH-sa-na*, Sanskrit – Ardha, half; Chandra, moon, glittering, shining)

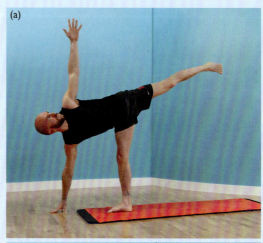

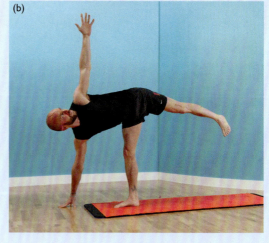

(a) Full position – leg straight, arm raised
(b) Modification – bent knee, small leg lift with arm raised

Purpose: A standing, balancing and lateral bending posture for strengthening and flexibility

Benefits:
- Strengthens the quadriceps, gluteals, abductors, gastrocnemius (supporting and lifted leg)
- Stretches adductors, hamstring, calf and hip flexor (both legs)
- Stretches pectorals and obliques
- Strengthens ankles
- Strengthens trunk and core muscles
- Improves balance, focus and concentration
- Mobility for hip, spine and shoulder
- Stimulates digestion
- Relieves stress

Suitable for: More advanced

Prohibitions:
- Mobility issues
- Arthritis in hip or hip replacement

Precautions:
- Vertigo, dizziness, pregnancy, high blood pressure, stay with Warrior 2 or triangle
- Limited range of motion: hand on blocks or chair, support knee can be bent and smaller leg raise

Instructions and teaching points:
- From Warrior 2
- Exhale
  - Lower the left (back) hand to left thigh
  - Hips and shoulders face forwards
  - Bend from hip and place right hand on the floor, six inches in front of right foot with weight on fingertips to support balance
  - Step the left foot backwards two paces
- Inhale
  - Shift the weight to the right (front) leg
  - Steadily lift the left (back) leg so that it is parallel to floor
  - Straighten right (front) knee, but keep knee unlocked
- Exhale
  - Raise the left arm (top) to ceiling, in line with right (lower) arm
  - Open the shoulder and chest, rotating left shoulder to back of room
  - Right hand can flatten to floor, if comfortable
  - Look forward
- Breathe comfortably while holding position

Progressions, modifications and variations:
- Modify to Warrior 2
- Hand can be supported on blocks or chair
- Lean against wall for balance

Visualisations:
- Feel the body opening and lengthening
- Crown of the head extends away from the base of the spine and legs
- Chest opens and focus point is the hand

Preparation: Warrior 2 or any modification listed

Counterpose: Opposite side

Figure 4.18 Revolved head to knee pose or Parivrtta Janu Sirsasana

(*Par-ee-vrt-tah Jaah-noo-sheer-SHAAH-sa-na,* Sanskrit – Parivrtta, revolved; Janu, knee; Shirsha, head)

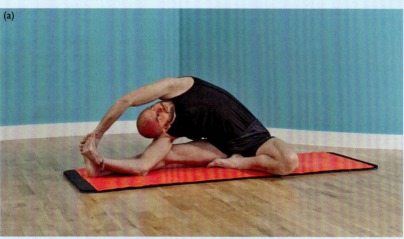

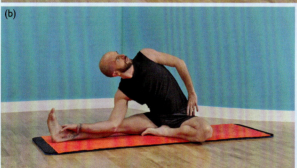

(a) Full position – hands hold feet and side bend
(b) Modification with hands on shin and small bend

Purpose: A seated side-bending posture

Benefits:
- Stretches hamstrings and gastrocnemius (straight leg)
- Stretches adductors (bent leg)
- Stretches erector spinae, obliques, latissimus dorsi
- Mobility for hip and spine
- Massages internal organs and stimulates digestion
- Promotes relaxation and relieves stress

Suitable for: All levels. Modifications can be used, as needed

Precautions:
- Lower back problems, sciatica: only move to a comfortable range of motion
- Low flexibility: use smaller range of motion, as illustrated
- Neck problem: look forward

Instructions and teaching points:
- Sitting in Dandasana (see page 122)
- Take right leg out to the side in a straddle position
- Bend the left leg and place the sole of the foot against the groin of right leg
- Inhale
  - Extend the left arm overhead
  - Shoulders away from ears
  - Abdominals engaged
  - Place right hand on right shin, as far down as is possible
- Exhale
  - Bend sideways and reach towards the right foot with the left hand
  - Lean directly to the side
  - Not leaning forwards or backwards
- Inhale
  - Reach right arm around ball of right foot
- Exhale
  - Lengthen further into stretch
  - Lowering left hand to reach right hand, around foot
  - Look upwards
- Breathe comfortably and hold position

Progressions, modifications and variations:
- Gentle side bend in sukhasana
- Seated on block
- Use belt around foot
- Hand stays at shin and reaches upwards
- A block or cushion can be placed under the knee of bent leg (if high)

Visualisations:
- Root chakra lengthens away from crown chakra
- Third eye chakra of forehead focuses towards ceiling
- Feel the vertebrae open and extend, unblocking any energy

Preparation: Seated side bend in sukhasana

Counterpose: Opposite side

STRENGTHENING POSTURES

Most yoga asanas challenge strength and balance. However, some do not neatly fit into the other categories, for example, they are not back bends or standing or seated. For this reason, the strengthening and balancing category has been added for fitness professionals. This category may not fit with traditional yoga thinking.

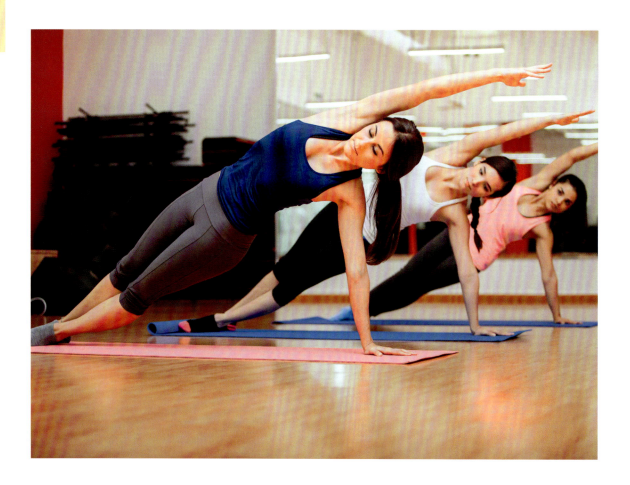

Figure 4.19 Plank or Khumbhakasana
(*Khum-baak-aasana*, Sanskrit – Khumbhak means to retain the breath)

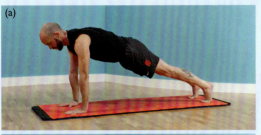
(a)

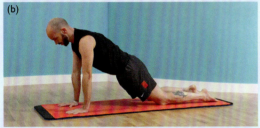
(b)

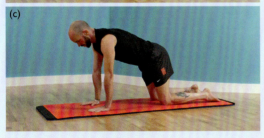
(c)

(a) Full position
(b) ¾ plank
(c) All fours

Purpose: A strengthening and balancing posture. It is one posture within the sun salutation – Surya Namaskara (sun salutations). The posture is a classic pose in a sun salutation where the breath is retained in the plank to create stability in the unusual plane of the body. It helps train the Hatha yogi in the art of breath retention in preparation for prananyama practices with breath retention.

Benefits:
- Strengthens biceps, triceps deltoids, trapezius, quadriceps, abductors, adductors, erector spinae, abdominals and core trunk stabiliser to hold position

Suitable for: Intermediate. Beginners use modifications

Prohibitions:
- Carpal tunnel syndrome
- Recurrent shoulder dislocation

Precautions:
- Wrist problems: can rest on fists, rather than spread hands
- Shoulder or lower back problems: use modifications
- Pregnancy: use modifications

Instructions and teaching points:
- From all fours
- Step right leg back with ball of the foot on the floor
- Engage abdominals
- Step left leg back
- Maintain spine alignment
- Elbows unlocked
- Breathe comfortably to hold position

Progressions, modifications and variations:
- All fours position
- Three-quarter position
- On elbows
- Hands or elbows on a step, chair or elevated bench to decrease range of motion

Visualisations:
- Maintain length and strength through the whole body

Preparation: Box position into single leg extension (both sides)

Counterpose: Child's pose (Balasana)

Figure 4.20 Four-limbed staff pose, crocodile pose or Chaturanga Dandasana

(*Chaht- tour-ANG-ah Don-DAH-sa-na*, Sanskrit – Chatur, four; anga, limb; Danda, staff or stick)

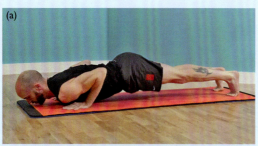

(a)

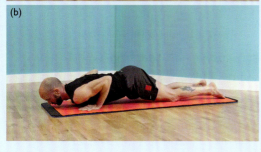

(b)

(a) Full position
(b) ¾ position

Purpose: A strengthening and balancing posture.

Benefits:
- Strengthens triceps and anterior deltoids
- Strengthens trapezius, gluteals, quadriceps, abductors, erector spinae, abdominals and core trunk stabiliser to hold position

Suitable for: Intermediate–advanced. Beginners use modifications

Prohibitions:
- Carpal tunnel syndrome
- Recurrent shoulder dislocation

Precautions:
- Wrist problems: can rest on fists, rather than spread hands
- Shoulder or lower back problems: use modifications
- Pregnancy: use modifications

Instructions and teaching points:
- From plank
- Maintain spine alignment
- Elbows into sides
- Bend elbows to point back to the feet and lower body
- Breathe comfortably to hold position

Progressions, modifications and variations:
- All fours lower and hold
- Three-quarter position lower and hold
- Hands on a step, chair or elevated bench to decrease range of motion

Visualisations:
- Maintain length and strength through the whole body
- Focus on the breath
- Body hovers over the earth
- Feel connection of groundedness

Preparation: Plank and modifications or three-quarter position

Counterpose: Child's pose (Balasana)

Figure 4.21 Side plank pose, T stand or Vasishthasana

(*Vas-eesht-AAH-sa-na*, Sanskrit – Vasishta, most excellent, best, richest)

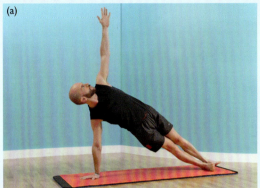

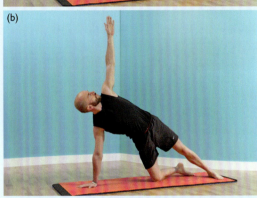

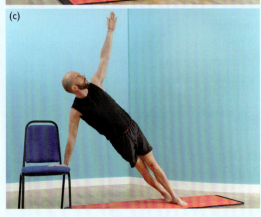

(a) Full position – Vasishthasana
(b) Modification – half side plank
(c) Modification on chair

Purpose: A lateral, balancing and strengthening posture

Benefits:
- Strengthens biceps, triceps deltoids, trapezius, quadriceps, abductors, adductors, erector spinae, abdominals and core trunk stabiliser
- Stretches pectorals and anterior deltoid
- Opens chest
- Improves balance and concentration

Suitable for: Intermediate. Beginners use modifications

Prohibitions:
- Carpal tunnel syndrome
- Recurrent shoulder dislocation
- Pregnancy after first trimester

Precautions:
- Wrist problems: can perform on elbows
- Low strength: kneeling variation

Instructions and teaching points:
- From all fours
- Keep the right knee under mid-line of body
- Left knee extends back, turning foot to a 90° angle and keeping foot flat on the floor
- Left hand moves to side of body, or hand on hip
- Rotate the body to face left (a quarter turn) keeping knee on floor (half plank)
- Transfer the weight to the right hand and left foot
- Lift the right knee and extend the leg, placing it behind the supporting left leg
- Inhale
  - Raise the left hand to ceiling and open the chest

- Breathe comfortably to hold the position
- Lower the body on an exhale

Progressions, modifications and variations:
- Kneeling version, see fig 4.19
- On elbows, see fig 4.19
- Hand or elbow on a step or chair to decrease range of motion

Visualisations:
- Open chest and heart chakra
- Throat chakra open
- Look upwards and focus to the top hand
- Feel strong and open

Preparation: Kneeling modification

Counterpose: Opposite side, rest in child's pose

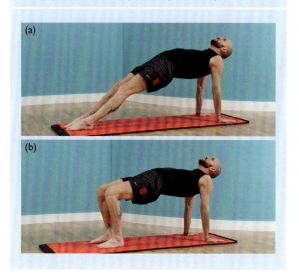

Figure 4.22 Upward-facing Plank, Intense East side stretch or Purvottanasana

(*Poohr-VHOT-Taahn-AAH-sa-na*, Sanskrit – Purva, East or front; uttana, Intense)

(a) Full position
(b) Modification – table

Purpose: A strengthening and extending posture. Counter posture for Paschimottanasana (forward bend)

Benefits:
- Strengthens gluteals, triceps, biceps, deltoids, erector spinae, sterno-cleido mastoid, gastrocnemius and hamstrings
- Strengthens wrist and forearm
- Stretches abdominals and anterior deltoid and pectorals

Suitable for: Intermediate. Beginners use modifications

Prohibitions:
- Carpal tunnel syndrome

- Recurrent shoulder dislocation
- Frozen shoulder

Precautions:
- Kyphosis, likely to lack flexibility in the chest: option to perform from step or bench with bent knees
- Pregnancy: use modifications
- Lower back problems: use modifications

Instructions and teaching points:
- From Dandasana or staff pose (see page 122)
- Inhale and raise the arms overhead and lengthen the spine
- Exhale and lower the arms and place hands on the floor about 12 inches away from buttocks, fingers point backwards
- Inhale
- Engage the abdominals and buttocks
- Elbows unlocked
- Lift body upwards and into a straight line, keeping toes on the floor (if possible)
- Shoulder away from ears, neck lengthened
- Breathe comfortably to hold position
- Exhale to lower

Progressions, modifications and variations:
- Bent leg variation – table top
- Perform on forearms with smaller lift
- Smaller range of motion (not lifting buttocks so high)
- Perform from step or bench to decrease range of motion

Visualisations:
- Throat chakra opens
- Feet strongly rooted to the floor

Preparation: Table top with bent knees

Counterpose: Seated forward bend or cross-legged forward bend

FORWARD-BENDING POSTURES

The forward-bending postures are those where the body is flexed from the hips with the spine straight or sometimes slightly rounding forward (but not bending from the waist). They include a range of both standing and seated positions, with the legs together or the legs open. The forward bends challenge flexibility, specifically of the hamstrings, gluteals and lower back. They also offer a massaging effect to the inner organs as the abdominal region contracts.

Figure 4.23 Standing forward bend or Uttanasana

(*Oot-taahn-AAH-sa-na*, Sanskrit – Ut, intense, deliberate; tana, stretch or lengthen)

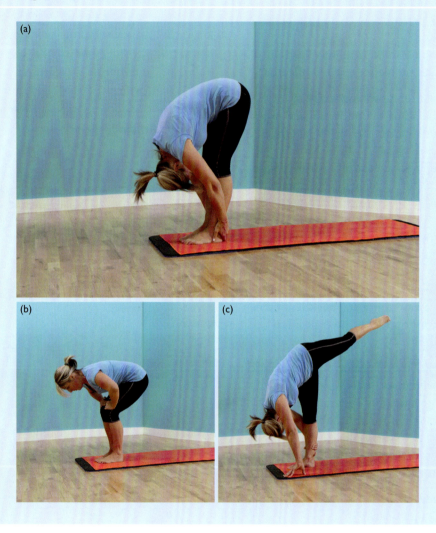

(a) Full position
(b) Modification: hands on thighs with knees bent
(c) Progression – standing split pose, Urdhva prasarita eka padasana, Upward, spread out, one, foot

Purpose: Standing, forward-bending posture (inversion), lengthening the spine and back of the thighs. It is one posture within the sun salutation – Surya Namaskara.

Benefits:
- Lengthens the hamstrings, gluteals, erector spinae and gastrocnemius muscles
- Strengthens quadriceps and abductors (holding position)
- Massages internal organs
- Increases blood flow to the brain
- Mobilises spine and hip
- Preparation for inversions
- Relieves mental and physical exhaustion
- Relieves indigestion

Suitable for: All levels. Use modified position for low flexibility

Prohibitions:
- Eye or ear problems, e.g. glaucoma
- High blood pressure: avoid dropping head
- Back injury or disc problems

Precautions:
- Knee hyperextension: keep knees unlocked
- Lower back pain: use modified position and move slower into and out of position
- Low blood pressure: move slowly into and out of position

Instructions and teaching points:
- From Tadasana
- Inhale
  - Raise arms overhead into prayer position
  - Shoulders away from ears
- Exhale
  - Hinge forward from the hips
  - Legs strong and straight, knees unlocked (modification: bend knees)
  - Crown of the head extends forward and down
  - Arms reach forward (diving) or can be extended at side of body or hands resting on hips/thighs
  - Lower hands to floor (if possible)
- Inhale
  - Relax spine and face
  - Awareness to balls of feet
- Exhale
  - Lengthen further into stretch and tuck head in
- Breathe comfortably
- For Pada Hastasana the index fingers are wrapped under and around the big toes with thumbs placed on top of the big toes

Progressions, modifications and variations:
- Knees bent and hands on thighs
- Knees bent and chest on thighs
- Knees bent and hands on floor
- Hands on to chair or wall or blocks
- Half forward bend – Ardha uttanasana (see page 96) with fingertips on floor, gazing forward and spine not tucking in towards thighs
- Can widen the leg position – see Prasarita padottanasana (see page 98)
- Take hands back further to floor at side of, or slightly behind, heels and tuck head in further
- Progress further by raising one leg upwards to the ceiling (standing split pose or Urdhva prasarita eka padasana – see page 96)

Visualisations:
- Crown of the head (crown chakra extends away)
- Chest to thigh to stimulate digestion
- Visualise the root chakra extending towards the ceiling

Preparation: Modified version with bent knees

Counterpose: Mountain pose (Tadasana) with small back bend

Figure 4.24 Wide-legged forward bend or Prasarita padottanasana

(*Pra-sa-ree-tah Pad-doh-tahn-Aah-sa-na*, Sanskrit – Prasarita, spread, expanded; pada, foot; ut, intense or deliberate; tan, stretch, extend)

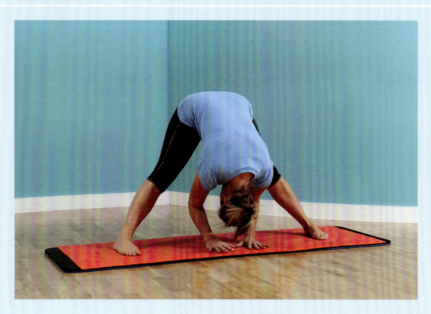

Purpose: Standing, forward-bending posture (inversion), lengthening the spine and back of the thighs

Benefits:
- Lengthens the hamstrings, gluteals, adductors, erector spinae and gastrocnemius muscles
- Strengthens quadriceps and abductors (holding position)
- Strengthens core trunk muscles to maintain spine alignment
- Open hip area
- Increase blood flow to the brain
- Mobilise spine and hip
- Preparation for inversions
- Relieves mental and physical exhaustion
- Relieves indigestion

Suitable for: All levels. Use modified positions, as needed

Prohibitions:
- Eye or ear problems, e.g. glaucoma
- High blood pressure: avoid dropping head
- Back injury or disc problems

Precautions:
- Knee hyperextension: keep knees unlocked
- Lower back pain: use modified position, with hands on chair or block, and move slower into and out of position
- Low blood pressure: move slowly into and out of position

Instructions and teaching points:
- From Tadasana
- Widen foot stance to about 3–4 feet apart
- Feet parallel and draw thighs upwards
- Inhale
  - Raise arms overhead into prayer position
  - Shoulders away from ears
- Exhale
  - Lower hands and place at side of hips/pelvis
  - Hinge forward from the hips
  - Gaze forward and keep spine long
  - Legs strong and straight, knees unlocked (modification – bend knees)
  - Crown of the head extends forward and down
  - Arms reach forward (diving) or can be extended at side of body or hands resting on hips/thighs
  - Lower fingertips to the floor
- Inhale
- Relax spine and face
- Exhale
  - Lengthen further into stretch
  - Bringing hands in closer and under hips, tuck head in
  - Bend elbows and lower forehead to floor (if possible)
- Breathe comfortably

Progressions, modifications and variations:
- Knees bent
- Hands on to chair or wall
- Hands can lower on to blocks
- Torso stays parallel, rather than fully bending forward
- Arms can reach forward (diving) from initial prayer position, rather than placing hands on hips
- Arms can be extended at side of body, like an aeroplane to lower into position

Visualisations:
- Crown of the head (crown chakra extends away)
- Chest to thigh to stimulate digestion
- Visualise the root chakra extending towards the ceiling

Preparation: Modified version with knees bent

Counterpose: Mountain pose (Tadasana) with small back bend

Figure 4.25 Same angle or Right angle posture or Samokonasana

(*Sam-o-kone-AAH-sa-na*, Sanskrit – Samo, same or equal; kona, angle, same/equal angle, or right angle)

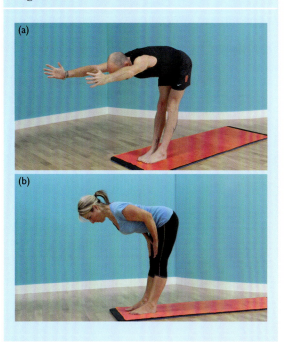

(a) Full position
(b) Modified version

Purpose: Strengthens the back and legs, and is a good preparation pose for standing forward bend (Uttanasana – see page 96)

Benefits:
- Strengthens back
- Mobility in hips
- Lengthens spine
- Stretches hamstrings
- Improves posture and spine alignment
- Strengthen core abdominal and spine muscles
- Improves digestion
- Assists calming of the mind ready for further practices

Suitable for: Supported – all levels; unsupported – experienced

Prohibitions: Lumbar spine issues

Precautions:
- Knee injury or hyperextension – knees should stay slightly bent
- Postural issues
- Vertigo

Instructions and teaching points:
- From Tadasana
- Inhale
  - Lengthen the spine
- Exhale
  - Flex forward from the hips to make a right angle with the chest to the floor
  - Keep the chest and back flat and parallel with chin tucked in with eye line to the floor
  - Stay for 3–12 breaths if holding or use in a vinyasa with equal breathing
- Inhale
  - Slowly come up to standing reaching the arms out and up
- Exhale
  - Float the arms back to the hips into Tadasana

Progressions, modifications and variations:
- One hand on one thigh with one arm extended (easier than full version)
- Bend the knees

Visualisations:
- Visualise a right angle with your legs and back in perfect alignment

Preparation: Chair

Counterpose: Forward bend followed by baby back bend

Figure 4.26 Single leg forward bend or Parsvottanasana

(*Paarsh-vot-taahn-AAH-sa-na*, Sanskrit – Parshva, side; ut, intense; tan, stretch)

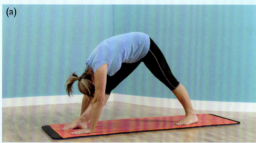
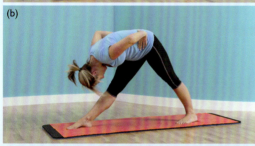
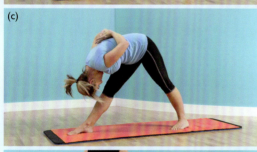
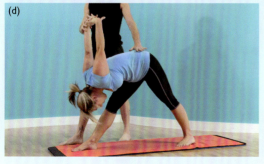

(a) Full position
(b) Hands on hips
(c) Hands in prayer
(d) Hands extended

Purpose: A standing forward bend; strengthening and stretching

Benefits:
- Strengthens the quadriceps and gluteals
- Stretches the hamstrings, gastrocnemius, hip flexor, adductors, anterior deltoid and pectorals
- Offers benefits of inversions
- Improves balance and concentration
- Mobility of hip, shoulder and spine
- Relieves stiffness in hip, shoulder, spine and wrist

Suitable for: Intermediate/advanced

Prohibitions:
- High blood pressure
- Ear and eye problems

Precautions:
- Shoulder mobility issues: hands on hips or isolate upper body stretches without forward bend
- Sciatica or lower back problems: bend to a 90° angle and use chair for support

Instructions and teaching points:
- Stand in Tadasana
- Widen feet to hip width
- Inhale
  - Step one leg backwards (about three feet), back foot turns slightly outwards
  - Both legs straight, weight spread equally between both feet
  - Clasp hands behind back and open chest
  - Shoulders away from ears
- Exhale
  - Bend from the hips and extend spine over thighs

- Keep abdominals engaged and spine lengthened
- Inhale
- Raise arms upwards, lengthening and opening chest
- Exhale
  - Bring the head towards the shin
  - Move deeper into stretch
- Breathe comfortably and hold position

Progressions, modifications and variations:
- Hands on hips
- Hands on chair to support body weight and lower back
- Narrower stance
- Front leg can be slightly bent
- Lengthen forward without dropping head
- Hands in prayer behind back
- Hands linked and extended behind back (Chest stretch position)

Preparation: Modified version

Counterpose: Opposite leg

Figure 4.27 Head to knee pose or Janu Sirsasana

(*Jaah-noo Sheer-SHAAH-sa-na*, Sanskrit – Janu, knee; Shirsha, head)

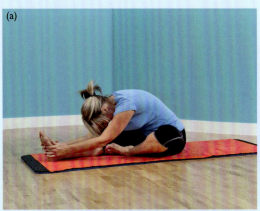

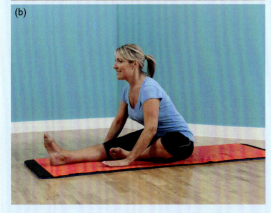

(a) Full position
(b) Modification – hands at side of shin, small bend and using block

Purpose: A seated forwards bending posture

Benefits:
- Stretches hamstrings, adductors, erector spinae, latissimus dorsi and gastrocnemius
- Mobility for hip and spine

- Massages internal organs and stimulates digestion
- Promotes relaxation and relieves stress

Suitable for: All levels. Modifications can be used, as needed

Prohibitions: Use modifications for any lower back problems, sciatica

Precautions:
- Lower back problems, sciatica: Only move to a comfortable range of motion
- Knee or hip problem: have knee slightly bent and in front of body, rather than tucking into thigh
- Pregnancy: adapt position to create space for bump

Instructions and teaching points:
- Sitting in Dandasana
- Bend the left leg and place the sole of the foot against the inner thigh of right leg
- Allow the hip to open and the bent leg to lower
- Inhale
  - Extend the arms overhead
  - Shoulders away from ears
  - Abdominals engaged
- Exhale
  - Bend forward from the hip and reach towards the right foot
  - Allow the chest and head to relax towards the knees
- Breathe comfortably and hold position

Progressions, modifications and variations:
- Seated on blocks
- Use belt around foot
- Hands at side of body and assist forward bend
- Hands level with knees and smaller bend
- Hands can wrap around feet
- Progress to Pashimottanasana (double leg forward bend)
- A block or cushion can be placed under the knee of bent leg (if high)

Visualisations:
- Feel the tail bone lengthen away from the crown of the head
- Root chakra lengthens away from crown chakra
- Third eye chakra of forehead focuses towards connection with the shin
- Feel the vertebrae open and extend, unblocking any energy

Preparation: With bent knees or smaller forward bend

Counterpose: Seated knees to chest (hug) followed by Small bridge or Upward-facing table top

Figure 4.28 Wide-angle seated forward bend or Upavistha Konasana

(*Oo-pah-VeeSH-ta Khon-AAH-sa-na*, Sanskrit – Upavista, seated; kona, angle)

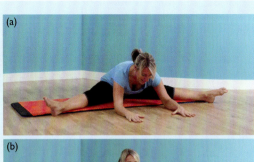

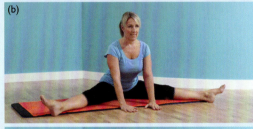

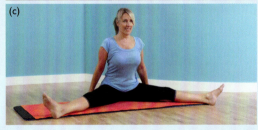

(a) Full position – chest on floor
(b) Modification – smaller bend – arms in front but not bent
(c) Urdhva konasana – wide leg stretch without forward bend

Purpose: A seated forward-bending and stretching posture

Benefits:
- Stretches adductors, hamstrings, gluteals, piriformis and erector spinae
- Core strengthening to hold spine in strong position
- Opens the hips and groin

Suitable for: More advanced. Other levels, use modifications

Precautions:
- Tight hips: use a narrower leg width
- Tight hamstrings of lower back: sit on block

Instructions and teaching points:
- Sit in Dandasana
- Inhale
  - Widen legs to side as far as is comfortable
- Exhale
  - Place hands in front of body on floor
  - Bend at hips (not the waist) and slide chest and arms forwards towards floor, head relaxed
  - Feet point towards ceiling
- Breathe comfortably and hold position

Progressions, modifications and variations:
- Narrower leg width
- Sit on blocks
- Hands supported at side of hip and without forward bend (Urdhva konasana)
- Smaller forward bend
- Viparita Kirani (a supine lying posture)

Visualisations:
- Feel the hips open
- Root chakra connects to the earth
- Crown chakra lengthens upwards
- Spine lengthens
- Breathe energy and strength into the body
- Breathe out any blocks or negative energies

Preparation: Dandasana, Narrow leg width and/or Sukhasana with forward bend

Counterpose: Belly twist

BACKWARD-BENDING POSTURES

The backward-bending postures are those which hyper-extend the spine. They develop strength and mobility of the muscles of the back and lengthen the abdominal muscle at the front of the trunk. Some also develop flexibility and strength of the upper body (e.g. wheel) and lengthening of other muscles (e.g. bow).

The back bends are often found to be the most challenging postures, which may be due to sedentary lifestyles, which promote a more flexed or flattened position and stiffness in the spine (e.g. sitting at desks, driving and hunched in chairs).

The back bends work intensely on the energy chakras that are located along the spine. They also open out the front of the body, which can give a psychological sense of expanding and opening, as many modern day activities, often close the body (e.g. hunching over a desk).

Figure 4.29 Bow pose or Dhanurasana
(*Dahn-oor-AAH-sa-na*, Sanskrit – Dhanu, bow)

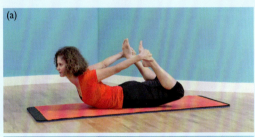
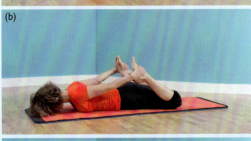
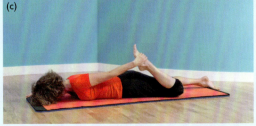

(a) Full position
(b) Double quad stretch without lift
(c) Single quad stretch as variation

Purpose: A back-bending posture. Mobility through spine extension and lengthening of abdominals and quadriceps

Benefits:
- Stretches the quadriceps, hip flexors, abdominals, pectorals and anterior deltoid
- Strengthens the gluteals, erector spinae, trapezius and rhomboids
- Spine mobility – hyperextension
- Opens the chest and hips
- Massages the abdominals
- Improves digestion
- Stimulates circulation to the abdominals and pelvic region

Suitable for: Intermediate. Beginners use modifications, as required

Prohibitions:
- Pregnancy
- Abdominal problems
- Hernia
- Heart problems
- Lower back problems

Precautions:
- Neck problems: look forward or block under forehead
- Lower back problems use smaller range of motion or modification (see below)
- Flat back or tight hips: rolled up mat or pillow under pubic bone and hips
- Lordosis: rolled up mat under pelvic bones (just below tummy button)

Instructions and teaching points:
- Lying on the front with arms at side of body
- Forehead on floor and chin tucked in
- Bend at knees and raise feet towards buttocks
- Hands take hold of the shins (or ankles if in reach)
- Inhale
- Raise the head and upper body away from the floor
- Exhale
- Raise the knees away from the floor and open knees slightly
- Body weight on the belly or tummy
- Elbows unlocked
- Breathe comfortably to hold position

Progressions, modifications and variations:
- Single leg quadriceps stretch
- Double leg quadriceps stretch
- Smaller lift with both legs
- Look down, rather than head looking forwards
- Cushion of mat under pelvic bones
- Straps to hold ankles

Visualisations:
- Visualise solar plexus chakra connecting with floor

Preparation: Single or double leg quad stretch

Counterpose: Child's pose or Cat

Figure 4.30 Cobra pose or Bhujangasana

(*Boo-jhang-AAH-sa-na*, Sanskrit – serpent)

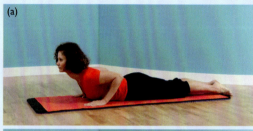

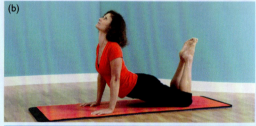

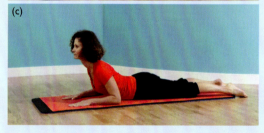

(a) Full position
(b) Progression – Cobra with knees bent and toes pointing towards ceiling
(c) Modification – Sphinx

Purpose: A back-bending posture. One posture within the sun salutation – Surya Namaskara

Benefits:
- Strengthen the erector spinae, gluteals, triceps and middle, lower trapezius
- Adductors strengthened to hold thighs together

- Stretches the abdominals and pectoralis and anterior deltoids
- Spine mobility
- Massages the abdominal region
- Promotes digestion and elimination
- Increases circulation to the abdomen and lungs

Suitable for: All levels. Beginners may need to use sphinx modification

Prohibitions:
- Pregnancy
- Abdominal problems
- Hernia
- Some back problems
- Carpal tunnel syndrome – use sphinx

Precautions:
- Lower back problems: smaller range of motion or sphinx, supported position
- Neck problems: look forward and/or include a neck rotation (right and left) at end of pose
- Winged scapula: draw scapula downwards and towards buttocks and ensure shoulders do not rise to ears, scrunching the neck

Instructions and teaching points:
- Lie on tummy
- Place hands by shoulders
- Lengthen neck
- Toes and heels together
- Inhale
  - Raise the chest off the floor
  - Elbows in
  - Shoulders away from ears
  - Hips on floor
- Exhale
  - Lower to resting position
- Or
  - Breathe comfortably to hold position

Progressions, modifications and variations:
- Sphinx with elbows on floor
- Progressively lift higher
- Upward dog
- Include neck rotation at end or use as an adaptation for kyphosis or for persons with neck shoulder tension

Visualisations:
- Crown chakra opens upwards
- Throat chakra opens
- Base and solar plexus chakra connected with the earth
- Feel the body opening

Preparation: Sphinx

Counterpose: Child's pose or Cat

Figure 4.31 Upward-facing dog pose or Urdhva Mukha Shvanasana

(*Urdh-va Muuk-ha Shvan-AAH-sa-na*, Sanskrit – Urdhva, rising upward; Mukha, face; Shvana, dog)

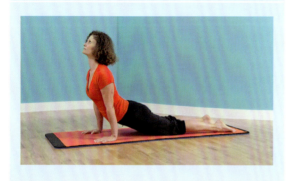

Purpose: A back-bending posture

Benefits:
- Strengthen the erector spinae, gluteals, triceps and middle, lower trapezius
- Stretches the abdominals and pectoralis and anterior deltoids
- Spine mobility
- Massages the abdominal region
- Promotes digestion and elimination
- Increases circulation to the abdomen and lungs

Suitable for: More advanced. Other levels use modifications

Prohibitions:
- Pregnancy
- Abdominal problems
- Hernia
- Some back problems
- Carpal tunnel syndrome – use sphinx

Precautions:
- Lower back problems: smaller range of motion or sphinx or cobra
- Neck problems: look forward and/or include a neck rotation (right and left) at end of pose
- Winged scapula: draw scapula downwards and towards buttocks and ensure shoulders do not rise to ears, scrunching the neck

Instructions and teaching points:
- Lie on tummy
- Place hands by shoulders, palms down
- Lengthen neck
- Toes and heels hip width apart
- Inhale
  - Connect with crown of head
  - Raise head and chest off the floor by pushing through hands
  - Elbows in
  - Shoulders away from ears
  - Chest open
  - Hips and thighs lift from floor
  - Lift onto the toes
  - Keep spine long
- Exhale
  - Lower to resting position
- Or
- Breathe comfortably to hold position

Progressions, modifications and variations:
- Sphinx
- Cobra
- Progressively lift higher

Visualisations:
- Throat chakra opens to look upwards

Preparation: Sphinx or Cobra

Counterpose: Child's pose, Cat or Downward-facing dog

Figure 4.32 Locust pose or Shalabasana

(*Shal-lahb-HAAH-sa-na*, Sanskrit – Shalaba, locust or grasshopper)

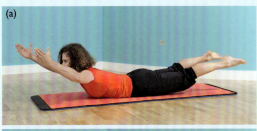

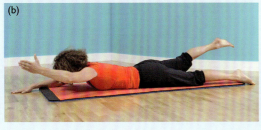

(a) Full position
(b) Modification single leg and arm

Purpose: An intense back-bending posture

Benefits:
- Strengthen the erector spinae, gluteals, triceps and middle, lower trapezius
- Stretches the abdominals and pectoralis and anterior deltoids
- Spine mobility
- Massages the abdominal region
- Promotes digestion and elimination
- Increases circulation to the abdomen and lungs

Suitable for: Advanced. Other levels can use modifications

Prohibitions:
- Pregnancy
- Abdominal problems
- Hernia
- Some back problems

Precautions:
- Lower back problems: use single leg lifts (see modifications)
- High blood pressure: use single leg modification

Instructions and teaching points:
- Lie on floor face down
- Feet in alignment with hips
- Forehead on floor and chin tucked in
- Arms by side and stretching to back corners of room
- Palms down
- Inhale
- Lift head and chest, maintaining alignment
- Exhale
- Lift both feet, arching the lower back
- Breathe deeply into the belly

Progressions, modifications and variations:
- Single leg (gluteal) raise and without body lift
- Opposite arm and leg raise
- Back raise keeping legs on floor (assisted with elbows on floor and progress to hands at side and hands side of head to increase weight lifted)
- Double arm lift only
- Double leg lift only

Preparation: Sphinx, or extension of legs and arms without lift; smaller lift

Counterpose: Child's pose, Cat or knees-to-chest (Apanasana)

Figure 4.33 Bridge pose (sometimes known as: Dwi Pada Pitham) or Setu Bandhasana

(*Sey-too Bahn-DHAA-sa-na*, Sanskrit – Setu, bridge or dam; bandha, lock)

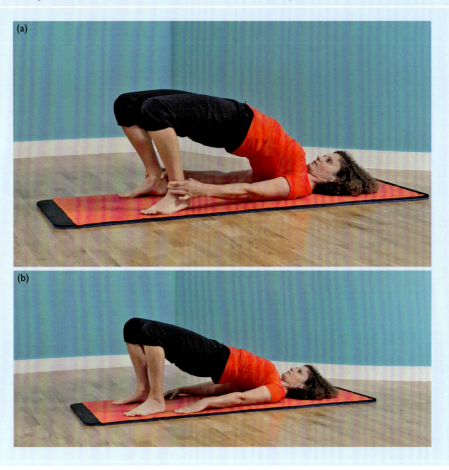

(a) Full position – holding ankles
(b) Modified – ROM

Purpose: A back-bending posture. Improves mobility through spine

Benefits:
- Strengthens quadriceps, gluteals, abductors and gastrocnemius
- Strengthens spine and core muscles
- Lengthens abdominals, pectorals and anterior deltoid
- Mobilises spine
- Opens hips and shoulders
- Increases circulation to thyroid
- Stimulates digestion
- Stimulates throat chakra
- Releases stress

Suitable for: All levels. Use modifications, as needed

Prohibitions:
- Pregnancy after first trimester
- Osteoporosis – use seated and gentle back bend

Precautions:
- Lower back pain: ensure gluteals activated and smaller lift or pelvic tilt
- Neck issues: smaller range of motion, not lifting fully onto shoulders
- Knee problems: smaller lift to decrease weight bearing

Instructions and teaching points:
- Lie supine on the back
- Knees bent and feet flat on the floor, behind buttocks
- Knees and ankles in line with hips
- Hands at side of body
- Lengthen and relax spine, neck and arms
- Keep shoulders away from ears, shoulder blades slide down towards buttocks
- Inhale
  - Activate gluteals and push equally through both feet
  - Raise hips upwards forming a bridge position
  - Push through arms to increase height of bridge and lift torso higher
- Exhale
  - Clasp hands underneath the body
  - Push the arms down towards the floor, elbows extended
  - Head and neck neutral
  - Breathe comfortably to hold position
- Lower body on an exhale

Progressions, modifications and variations:
- Activate gluteals and small pelvic tilt
- Feet further away from buttocks
- Small lift, progress to higher lift
- Block between knees to prevent knees opening outwards
- Hands on lower back to create larger back bend
- Hands reach to hold ankles
- In position, option to raise one leg to ceiling

Visualisations:
- At top of movement, focus on hearing the breath and activating throat chakra
- Breathe deeply and widely into ribcage and abdomen

Preparation: Smaller lift

Counterpose: Knees-to-chest (Apanasana)

Figure 4.34 Camel pose or Ustrasana
(*Oosh-TRAAH-sa-na*, Sanskrit – Ustra, camel)

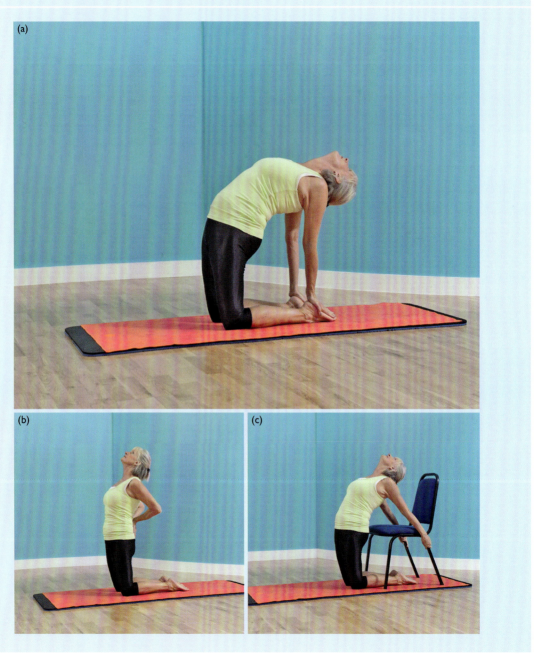

(a) Full position
(b) Modification with hands on lower back and smaller bend
(c) Full position using a stool or step to support body

Purpose: A back-bending posture

Benefits:
- Stretches quadriceps, hip flexors, abdominals, pectoralis, anterior deltoid and sterno cleido-mastoid
- Strengthens gluteals and abductors to hold position
- Mobilises the spine
- Opens hips and chest
- Stretches the front of the neck and opens the throat chakra region
- Stimulates thyroid

Suitable for: Intermediate. Beginners use modifications

Prohibitions: Use modifications for back problems/balance issues

Precautions:
- Any mobility problems or stiffness in hips, shoulder, spine and wrist: use modified version
- Neck problems or vertigo: avoid dropping head back
- Kneeling discomfort: place blanket under knees
- Back problems: use modified version

Instructions and teaching points:
- Kneel with feet and knees together, sitting on heels
- Lift buttocks away from heels, buttocks in line with knees and spine aligned
- Arms at the side of the body (or on hips for modification)
- Right hand reaches for right heel, without strain
- Left hand reaches for left heel, without strain
- Arch backwards opening the spine and press hips forward
- Shoulder away from ears
- Gently arch the neck to look upwards
- Weight is spread equally through arms and legs
- Breathe comfortably to hold position

Progressions, modifications and variations:
- Hands on hips, without bend
- Hands on hips and small bend
- Use a stool or small bench/step (level to hip height) to support body
- Hands on block behind body, rather than on floor or holding feet
- Hips face wall and press towards wall to open the hips

Visualisations:
- Throat chakra opens
- Third eye chakra connects upwards

Preparation: Hands on buttocks and small backward bend

Counterpose: Child's pose

Figure 4.35 Wheel pose or Chakrasana, also known as Upward-facing bow (*Chak-RAAH-sa-na*, Sanskrit – Chakra, wheel or vortex; Urdhva, upward; Dhana, bow)

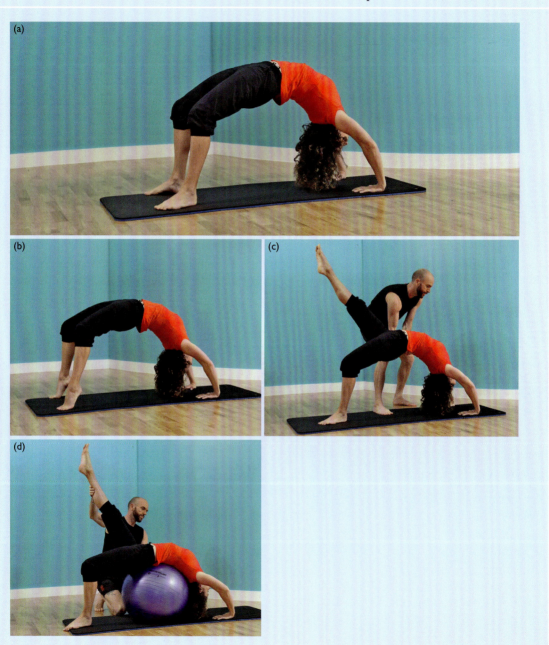

(a) Full position
(b) Full position with heels lifted
(c) Full position with leg raised and assistance
(d) Modification using ball

Purpose: A strong back-bending posture

Benefits:
- Stretches quadriceps, hip flexors, abdominals, pectoralis, biceps, anterior deltoid
- Strengthens gluteals and abductors, gastrocnemius, upper trapezius, triceps, medial deltoid and rhomboids to hold position
- Mobilises the spine, shoulder, elbows and hips
- Stretches and opens the front of the body
- Stimulating for thyroid, pineal and pituitary glands

Suitable for: Advanced

Prohibitions:
- Back and spine conditions
- Osteoporosis
- High blood pressure
- Pregnancy
- Abdominal surgery
- Heart or cardiac conditions
- Carpal tunnel syndrome or wrist problems
- Vertigo or dizziness

Precautions: An advanced back-bending position. Modification can be used by healthy persons to build into position

Instructions and teaching points:
- Lie supine, on the back with knees bent and heels close to buttocks at hip width
- Reach the hands upwards and overhead, bending the elbows and lower hands to the floor at side of ears, with fingertips facing body
- Push evenly through the feet and hands and lift the body and head away from the floor
- Create an arching shape of the torso at the top of the movement
- Relax the face and neck
- Breathe comfortably to hold position

Progressions, modifications and variations:
- Modification: perform lying on a step/bench to decrease range of motion and offer support to the body
- Modification: perform using a stability ball
- Progression: rise on to balls of feet at the top of the movement
- Progression: raise one leg to ceiling at top of the movement

Visualisations:
- Become the wheel
- Open the chest and front of the body in an arc
- Feel all the chakras of the spine become exposed to the universal life-force

Preparation: Shoulder bridge

Counterpose: Knees-to-chest (Apanasana)

Figure 4.36 Fish pose or Matsyasana
(*Maht-see-YAH-sa-na*, Sanskrit – Matsya, fish)

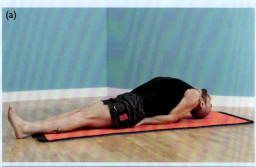

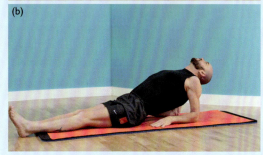

(a) Full position
(b) Half fish

Purpose: A back-bending posture

Benefits:
- Stretches the abdominals, pectorals and anterior deltoid
- Strengthens the deltoids, triceps and biceps to hold position
- Opens the chest, shoulders and throat
- Aids respiratory ailments

Suitable for: Intermediate

Prohibitions:
- Shoulder or neck injuries
- High blood pressure
- Back problems

Precautions:
- Vertigo or dizziness: avoid lowering the head

Instructions and teaching points:
- Lie in a supine position
- Place the hands under the buttocks, palms face floor
- Elbows as close together as possible
- Lengthen neck, drawing shoulders away from ears
- Legs together but relaxed
- Inhale
  - Lift onto elbows, raising chest upwards
  - Forearms flat
  - Arch the back and lower crown of head towards the floor
- Exhale
  - Relax into position
  - Breathe comfortably and deeply to hold position
- Lower on an exhale

Progressions, modifications and variations:
- Perform without lowering head
- Lie over a step with blankets to support back in arched position

Visualisations:
- Draw your elbows close together like a bow to expand the chest as far as possible
- Imagine floating on a lake while breathing slowly and fully

Preparation: Resting on elbows without backward bend, or head lower

Counterpose: Knees-to-chest (Apanasana)

SEATED ASANAS

The seated postures work on opening up the hip, knee and ankle joints and groin area. They lengthen the spine and demand strength from the core muscle to maintain an upright position.

Psychologically, the seated postures are ideal for practising meditation and pranayama, and promoting stillness in the body and mind, and connection and focus on the breath.

Figure 4.37 Easy pose, Cross-legged pose or Sukhasana

(*Sook-AAH-sa-na*, Sanskrit – Sukh, joy or comfort)

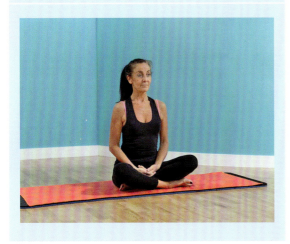

Purpose: Seated posture that can be used for meditation and chanting. Can also be used for seated mobility during preparation phase and pranayama exercises during closing phase

Benefits:
- Opens hips
- Stretches adductors
- Strengthens erector spinae and core abdominals
- Improves seated posture
- Relieves stress

Suitable for: All levels

Precautions:
- Knee injury: legs not so tightly crossed or straighten one or both legs
- Tight hips and back: sit on block or sit with back against wall
- Long coccyx or tail bone or bony bottom: sit on a cushion

Instructions and teaching points:
- Sit in a cross-legged position
- Lengthen spine
- Breathe

Progressions, modifications and variations:
- Siddhasana (Perfect pose)
- Ardha Padmasana (Half lotus)
- Padmasana (Lotus)
- Hands can be placed in chin mudhra by knees
- Hands can be placed in prayer position by chest
- Palms can rest on top of each other in lap

Visualisations
- Root chakra connects with floor
- Crown chakra extends to ceiling
- Feel a balanced flow of upwards and downwards energy
- Heart chakra open

Figure 4.38 Adept pose, Perfect pose or Siddhasana
(*Sid-HAA-sa-na*, Sanskrit – Siddha, perfect, content or adept)

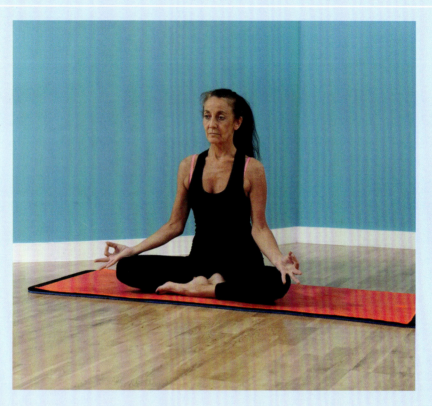

Purpose: Seated posture that can be used for meditation and chanting. Can also be used for seated mobility during preparation phase and pranayama exercises during closing phase

Benefits:
- Opens hips
- Stretches adductors
- Strengthens erector spinae and core abdominals
- Improves seated posture
- Relieves stress
- Channels prana towards third eye chakra (Ajna chakra)
- Lowers heart rate and blood pressure

Suitable for: Advanced. Other levels use modifications, as necessary

Precautions:
- Tight hips: use Sukhasana and place blocks under knees if necessary
- Knee injuries: use wide-legged position

Instructions and teaching points:

Men	Women
Sitting on sitting bones	Sitting on sitting bones
Legs in straddle/wide position	Legs in straddle wide position
Bend and cross LEFT heel into perineum	Bend and cross RIGHT heel into vagina
Bend and cross RIGHT in front (presses on pubic bone, above genitals)	Bend and cross LEFT in front (presses on pubic bone, clitoris)
Knees as close to floor as possible	Knees as close to floor as possible
Lengthen spine	Lengthen spine
Crown of head lengthens towards ceiling OR	Crown of head lengthens towards ceiling OR
Relax head and lower chin towards collarbone, gazing into third eye chakra between eyebrows	Relax head and lower chin towards collarbone, gazing into third eye chakra between eyebrows

The *Hatha Yoga Pradipka* indicates that siddhasana can only be practised by men and the equivalent posture for women is: *Siddha yoni asana*; where the lower heel presses against the vagina and top heel presses against the clitoris.
(Swami Muktibodhananda, *HYP*, 1993:104)

Visualisations
- Root chakra connects with floor
- Crown chakra extends to ceiling
- Feel a balanced flow of upwards and downwards energy
- Heart chakra open
- Hands can be positioned in prayer position at chest
- Hands positioned using chin mudra (see page 164)

The *Hatha Yoga Pradipika* indicates that *'if one can master this asana one will acquire siddhis'*
(Swami Muktibodhananda, *HYP*, 1993:105)

Preparation: Cross-legged (Sukhasana)

Counterpose: Corpse

Progressions, modifications and variations:
- Sit on a block
- Sukhasana
- Ardha padmasana – half lotus
- Padmasana – full lotus
- Wide-legged position

Figure 4.39 Half lotus pose or Ardha padmasana

(*Are-dah Pahd-MAHS-anna*, Sanskrit – Ardha, half; Padma, lotus)

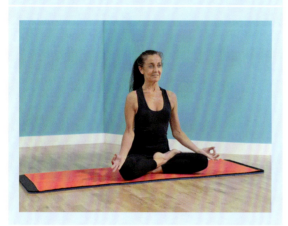

Purpose: Seated posture that can be used for meditation and chanting and pranayama

Benefits:
- Opens hips
- Stretches adductors
- Strengthens erector spinae and core abdominals
- Improves seated posture
- Stretches ankles
- Relieves stress

Suitable for: Advanced. Other levels use modifications, as necessary

Prohibitions:
- Knee injury
- Ankle injury

Precautions:
- Tight hips: use sukhasana and place blocks under knees if necessary

Instructions and teaching points:
- Sitting on sitting bones
- Legs wide
- Right foot crosses on top of left thigh with heels pressed against groin
- Left foot crosses in, but under right thigh
- Lengthen spine
- Crown of head lengthens towards ceiling

Progressions, modifications and variations:
- Sit on block
- Use block to support knees
- Sukhasana
- Siddhasana

Visualisations:
- Root chakra connects with floor
- Crown chakra extends to ceiling
- Feel a balanced flow of upwards and downwards energy
- Hands positioned using chin mudra (see page 164)

Preparation: Cross-legged (Sukhasana)

Counterpose: Other side (switch legs) and then staff pose (Dandasana)

Figure 4.40 Lotus pose or Padmasana

(*Pahd-MAHS-anna*, Sanskrit – Padma, lotus)

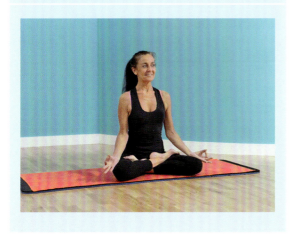

Purpose: Seated posture that can be used for meditation and chanting and pranayama

The yogi who sits in Padmasana and holds the breath inhaled through both nadis is liberated without a doubt
(*Hatha Yoga Pradipika*, Chapter 1. Verse 49).

Benefits:
- Opens hips
- Stretches adductors
- Strengthens erector spinae and core abdominals
- Improves seated posture
- Stretches ankles
- Relieves stress

Suitable for: Advanced. Other levels use modifications, as necessary

Prohibitions:
- Knee injury
- Ankle injury
- Varicose veins

Precautions:
- Tight hips: use sukhasana and place blocks under knees if necessary

Instructions and teaching points:
- From wide-legged seated position
- Bend right foot to cross over left thigh
- Bend left foot to cross over right thigh
- Lengthen spine
- Hands in chin mudra

Progressions, modifications and variations:
- Sit on block
- Use block to support knees
- Sukhasana
- Siddhasana

Visualisations:
- Root chakra connects with floor
- Crown chakra extends to ceiling
- Feel a balanced flow of upwards and downwards energy
- Heart chakra open
- Hands can be in prayer position at chest
- Hands positioned using chin mudra (see page 164)

Preparation: Cross-legged (Sukhasana) or half lotus

Counterpose: Other side (switch legs) and then staff pose (Dandasana)

Figure 4.41 Staff pose or Dandasana
(*Dan-DAHH-sa-na*, Sanskrit – Danda, staff or walking stick)

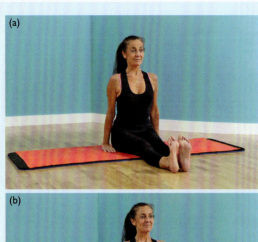

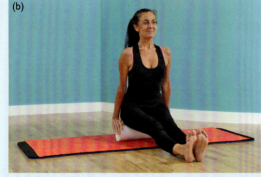

(a) Full position
(b) Modification – seated on blocks

Purpose: Seated posture which offers the foundation for other seated postures

Benefits:
- Lengthens gluteals, hamstrings and erector spinae
- Strengthens core muscle of the trunk
- Improves seated posture
- Improves postural awareness
- Enhances emotional stability
- Assists breathing (open posture)

Suitable for: All levels

Precautions:
- Lower back pain: can sit with back against wall

Instructions and teaching points:
- Sit upright on the sitting bones with both legs extended forward, toes upwards
- Lift the fat of the buttocks with your hands to achieve full sitting bone position
- Body at right angle
- Palms on floor at side of hips and lengthen upwards
- Elbows and knees unlocked
- Lengthen spine, engage abdominals
- Chin parallel
- Crown of head extends upwards
- Shoulders slide down towards buttocks
- Breathe comfortably and hold position

Progressions, modifications and variations:
- Seated on blocks to reduce range of motion
- Hands on blocks if necessary
- Slight knee bend for thigh hamstrings
- Sit against wall for back support

Visualisations:
- Root chakra grounded to floor
- Crown chakra extends to ceiling
- Lengthen the spine
- Breathe wide into ribcage
- Feel energy flowing down and up spine on inhale and exhale
- Allow the mind to settle

Preparation: Smaller range of motion, upright seated position with hands supporting body further back or knees slightly bent

Counterpose: Wind-relieving pose (Apanasana)

Figure 4.42 Boat pose or Navasana

(*Nav-AAH-sa-na*, Sanskrit – Nava, boat or ship)

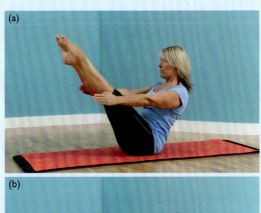

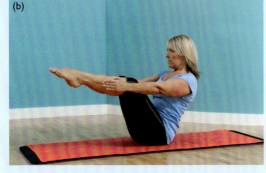

(a) Full position – legs straight, arms extended
(b) Modification – bend knees

Purpose: A seated balancing posture

Benefits:
- Strengthens core muscle of trunk
- Strengthens quadriceps and hip flexors
- Stretches hamstrings (when legs extended)
- Strengthen deltoids and upper trapezius when arms elevated
- Massages internal organs, stimulates digestion
- Improves balance and concentration

Suitable for: All levels, use modified position for beginners

Prohibitions:
- Lower back problems
- Pregnancy

Precautions:
- Mild lower back pain: use modified position
- Weaker core muscles: use modified position

Instructions and teaching points:
- Sit in Dandasana
- Inhale
  - Place hands behind the back for support
  - Lean back from the hips (about a 45° angle)
- Exhale
  - Engage abdominals
  - Raise the feet away from the floor, knees bent initially, creating a 45° angle at hip
  - Extend the legs straight, creating a 'V' shape (option to move one leg at a time)
- Inhale
  - Prepare for balance and focus
- Exhale
  - Raise arms straight in front and level with the shins (option to hold thighs or calves)
- Breathe comfortably and hold position

Progressions, modifications and variations:
- Single leg and arm (opposing) with knee bent
- Bend knees to reduce lever length and resistance held
- Hands behind back for support
- Hands can hold legs for support
- Feet on stability ball or chair
- Sit on cushion (individuals with a bony coccyx)
- Sit on stability pad to challenge balance

Visualisations:
- Create the 'V' shape of a boat's hull

Preparation: Dandasana and modified boat

Counterpose: Bridge or wind-relieving pose (Apanasana)

Figure 4.43 Cobbler's pose or Baddhakonasana

(*Bhaad-dah-kohn-AAH-sa-na*, Sanskrit – Baddha, bound or caught; Kona, angle)

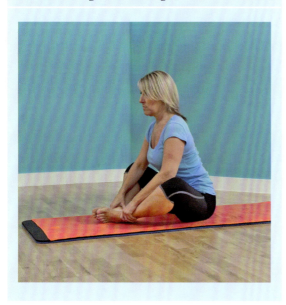

Purpose: A seated posture that stretches the inner thigh

Benefits:
- Stretches adductors
- Strengthens core abdominal and back muscles
- Promotes improved posture
- Opens the hips
- Helps to relieve sacroiliac pain and discomfort
- Reduces sciatic pain

Suitable for: All levels. Modify, as needed

Precautions:
- Tight hips: blocks under knees
- Tight hamstrings or lower back or flat back posture: use block under buttocks or sit with back against a wall

Instructions and teaching points:
- From Dandasana
- Sit up tall on the sitting bones, use hand behind back to lift upwards
- Bend the knees to crook seated position, feet on floor, ankles together
- Allow the hips to open, so that knees move towards the floor, soles of feet together
- Hands can be used to help draw feet inwards
- Heels into perineum
- Draw the trunk upwards
- Pivot slightly forwards from the hips
- Breathe comfortably to hold position

Progressions, modifications and variations:
- Sit on a block
- Sit with back against wall and hold ankles
- Supine lying version
- One leg straight and one bent
- Progress to Upavistha Konasana – Wide angle seated forward bend

Visualisations:
- This posture is so called because traditional cobblers in India sat in this position to repair and make shoes

Preparation: Cross-legged (Sukhasana)

Counterpose: Staff pose (Dandasana)

Figure 4.44 Hero pose or Virasana/Vajrasana

(*Va-RAAH-sa-na*, Sanskrit – Vira, hero, chief or warrior)

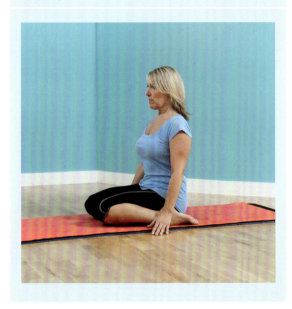

Purpose: A seated posture. Can be used for meditation as a preparation or modification for other kneeling postures. Counterpose for hip opening postures (e.g. lotus)

Benefits:
- Stretches quadriceps and tibialis anterior
- Stretches ankles
- Mobility in hips and knees
- Improves posture and spine alignment
- Strengthen core abdominal and spine muscles
- Improves digestion
- Assists calming of the mind ready for meditation

Suitable for: All levels

Prohibitions:
- Knee surgery replacement

Precautions:
- Knee injury or tight quadriceps: place block between buttocks and heels
- Ankle injury: cushion under ankles

Instructions and teaching points:
- Kneeling on the floor
- Take feet outside of buttocks, keep knees together
- Use hands to roll calf muscle outside of thighs
- Toes point backwards
- Spine lengthened and chest open
- Breathe comfortably to hold position

Progressions, modifications and variations:
- Block between buttocks and heels
- Buttocks on heels
- Cushion under ankles
- Progress to reclining hero

Visualisations:
- Imagine the shape of a bolt of lightning

Preparation: Modified hero with buttocks resting on heels

Counterpose: Sphinx or prone lying

Figure 4.45 Side twist in the Hero pose or Parsva Virasana

(*Pah-svah Va-RAAH-sa-na*, Sanskrit – Parsva, side or flank; Vira, hero, chief or warrior)

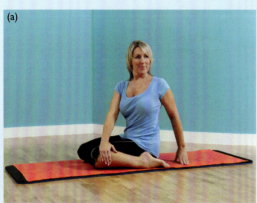

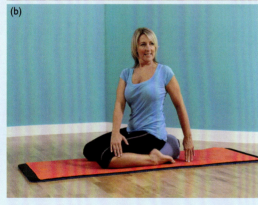

(a) Full position
(b) Modification using cushions

Purpose: A seated posture. Can be used as part of preparation and closing phases of the session

Benefits:
- Stretches quadriceps and tibialis anterior
- Stretches ankles
- Mobility in hips and knees
- Mobilises spine
- Stretches obliques
- Improves posture and spine alignment
- Strengthen core abdominal and spine muscles
- Improves digestion
- Assists calming of the mind ready for meditation

Suitable for: All levels

Prohibitions:
- Knee surgery replacement

Precautions:
- Knee injury or tight quadriceps: place block between buttocks and heels
- Ankle injury: cushion under ankles

Instructions and teaching points:
- From hero
- Inhale
  - Lengthen the spine
- Exhale
  - Rotate spine to the right and look right
- Inhale
  - Return to centre
- Exhale
  - Rotate spine to the left and look left
- Inhale
- Return to centre

Progressions, modifications and variations:
- Block between buttocks and heels
- Cushion under ankles

Visualisations:
- Twist the body like a damp cloth being wrung out

Preparation: Hero

Counterpose: Opposite side

Figure 4.46 Downward-facing Hero pose or Adhomukha Virasana

(*Arr-do-Moo-ka Va-RAAH-sa-na*, Sanskrit – Adho, downwards; Mukha, face; Vira, hero, chief or warrior)

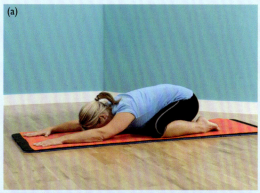
(a)

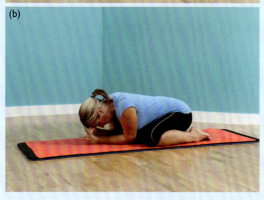
(b)

(a) Full position
(b) Modification with hands under forehead

Purpose: A seated posture. Can be used for relaxation

Benefits:
- Stretches quadriceps and tibialis anterior and erector spinae and latissimus dorsi
- Stretches ankles
- Mobility in hips and knees and spine
- Improves digestion
- Assists calming of the mind
- Rejuvenating when tired
- Relieves breathlessness
- De-stresses and calms the body

Suitable for: All levels

Prohibitions:
- Knee surgery replacement

Precautions:
- Knee injury or tight quadriceps: place block between buttocks and heels
- Ankle injury: cushion under ankles
- Kyphosis: block under forehead

Instructions and teaching points:
- From kneeling hero
- Place hands on thighs
- Slide hands forward until chest rests on thighs, forehead on floor
- Arms extended and shoulders away from ears
- Breathe comfortably to hold position

Progressions, modifications and variations:
- Block between buttocks and heels
- Cushion under ankles
- Block under forehead

Visualisations:
- Solar plexus and heart chakra connect with thigh
- Surrender the upper body to the lower body
- Third eye chakra connects to the floor

Preparation: Hero

Counterpose: Corpse, sphinx or wind-relieving pose (Apanasana)

Figure 4.47 Reclined hero pose, or Supta virasana

(*Soopta Va-RAAH-sa-na*, Sanskrit – Supta, reclined, lying down; Vira, hero, chief or warrior)

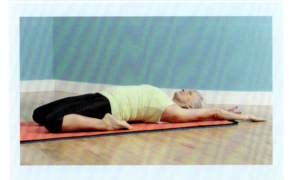

Instructions and teaching points:
- From Hero position
- Ankles outside of buttocks
- Keep spine long
- Lean backwards and take weight backwards onto elbows
- Steadily lower whole body to the floor
- Breathe comfortably to hold position

Progressions, modifications and variations:
- Bolster underneath back to reduce range of motion
- Head can rest on pillow
- Kneeling variation

Preparation: Hero

Counterpose: Wind-relieving pose (Apanasana)

Purpose: Intense stretching posture

Benefits:
- Stretches quadriceps, hip flexor and tibialis anterior
- Stretches ankles
- Mobility in hips and knees and ankles
- Can promote relaxation
- Tones pelvic organs
- Relieves indigestion
- Increase elasticity of lung tissue
- Helps to correct flat feet

Suitable for: Advanced

Prohibitions:
- Knee surgery replacement
- Lower back problems, sciatica

Precautions:
- Knee injury or tight quadriceps: use kneeling version
- Ankle injury: cushion under ankles

Figure 4.48 Marichi's pose, Sage's pose or Marichyasana

(*Mar-ee-chee-AAH-sa-na*, Sanskrit – Marichi, ray of light)

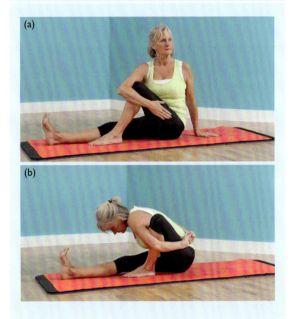

(a) Full centre fold position
(b) Progression with arms wrapped behind back

Purpose: A seated and twisting posture

Benefits:
- Stretches obliques and abductors
- Opens chest and shoulders
- Mobilises spine and hip
- Improves seated posture
- Strengthens abdominals and core muscles
- Massages internal organs
- Rotations wring out tension from body
- Removes toxins from internal organs
- Rejuvenates the body

Suitable for: Beginner (arm wrapping, listed in variations and illustrated is for advanced level)

Prohibitions:
- Pregnancy
- Hernia

Precautions:
- Lower back problems: can twist away from bent leg
- Neck problems: look forward
- Hip problems: sit on a block
- Flat back or tightness in back or hip: can sit against a wall for support
- Kyphosis: focus on sitting upright

Instructions and teaching points:
- From Dandasana or Staff pose
- Bend right knee and place foot flat on the floor
- Inhale
  - Sit upright and lengthen the body
  - Take right hand on the floor about a foot away from buttocks, fingers point backwards
  - Take left elbow to outside of right knee
- Exhale
  - Rotate to the right leaning slightly backwards during rotation, to increase twisting action
  - Look behind and over right shoulder
- Breathe comfortably to hold position
- Return to Dandasana on an inhale

Progressions, modifications and variations:
- Use hands to bring knee to chest and small rotation
- Twist away from bent leg
- Sit on a block or small step/bench
- Progress to Ardha Matsyendrasana or Half lord of the fishes
- Hands can link behind the back (as illustrated)

Visualisations: Imagine you are tight and constricted and let the breathing rate relax

Preparation: Dandasana

Counterpose: Opposite side, wind-relieving pose (Apanasana)

Figure 4.49 Lion pose or Simhasana
(*Sim-HAA-sa-na*, Sanskrit – Sima, lion)

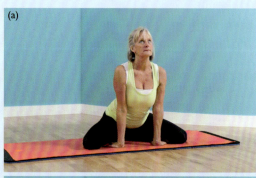
(a)

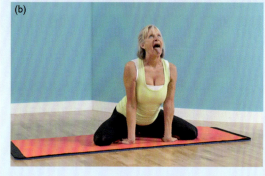
(b)

(a) Lion
(b) Roaring lion

Purpose: Back-bending posture, can be used for meditation

Benefits:
- Stretches quadriceps and tibialis anterior and pectoralis and anterior deltoids
- Stretches ankles
- Mobility in hips and knees and spine
- Opens chest and shoulders
- Stimulating

Suitable for: All levels

Precautions:
- Knee injury or tight quadriceps: place block between buttocks and heels
- Ankle injury: cushion under ankles
- Neck problems: look forward
- Wrist injury: hands on thighs

Instructions and teaching points:
- From hero, kneeling on the floor
- Open the knees to a wide and comfortable position
- Toes touching
- Lean forwards
- Place the hands on the floor, palms flat with fingers facing body
- Keep the arms straight, elbows unlocked
- Arch the back
- Gently tilt the head backwards, opening throat chakra, to feel a gentle tension
- Close the eyes and focus on the third eye chakra (between eyebrows)
- Breathe comfortably to hold position for meditation

Progressions, modifications and variations:
- Block between buttocks and heels
- Hands on thighs
- Look forward if neck problems
- Cushion under ankles
- Roaring lion as variation, with mouth open

Visualisations:
- Throat chakra opens
- Visualise self as a lion in waiting

Preparation: Hero

Counterpose: Child's pose

Figure 4.50 Cow face posture or Gomukasana

(*Go-mook AAH-sa-na*, Sanskrit – Go, cow; mukha, face)

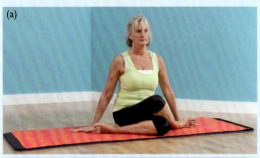

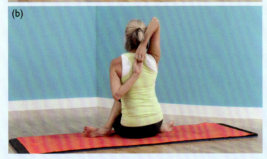

(a) Front view
(b) Rear view

Purpose: A seated stretching posture

Benefits:
- Stretches pectorals, anterior deltoid and triceps
- Opens shoulders and chest
- Mobility for shoulder, elbow, wrist and spine
- Massages internal organs
- Stimulates digestion

Suitable for: Intermediate. Use modifications, as needed

Prohibitions:
- Frozen shoulder or other shoulder injuries

Precautions:
- Knee problems: use hero position, with cushions under buttocks and without forward bend
- Limited shoulder mobility: use towel or strap instead of clasping hands
- Back problems: no forward lean

Instructions and teaching points:
- From seated and cross-legged position
- Cross the right foot further over the left thigh, with one knee stacked on top of the other
- Feet point outwards, same distance from hips
- Can use hands to draw the ankles forwards
- Lower buttocks to the floor
- Look forward, with space between shoulders and ears
- Crown of the head extends upwards
- Reach right arm up to ceiling and lower hand to between shoulder blades
- Left arm reaches behind and elbow bends to reach right hand
- Hands clasped (or use towel or strap)
- Hold position, breathing comfortably OR
- Bend forward from the hip and bring head towards knee

Progressions, modifications and variations:
- Use strap to assist hand grip
- Stay upright seated, without forward bend
- Isolate arm movement, could perform standing or chair seated
- Isolate leg action
- Ankles closer to buttock
- Blanket or blocks under buttocks

Visualisations:
- Crown chakra lengthens towards ceiling
- Root chakra connected with floor

Preparation: Hero

Counterpose: Child's pose (Balasana)

SUPINE LYING ASANAS

The reclining or lying postures are those where the body is most supported and restful. They are the postures used for relaxation at the beginning and end of a yoga session.

The lying postures allow stillness and promote non-movement and relaxation of the muscles. They are ideal for focusing on pranayama and deeper breathing and give the body time to rest and recover.

Psychologically, the lying postures give space to release and let go of physical and mental tension and create a sense of calm and peace, which, in turn, can help to give a renewed energy and confidence.

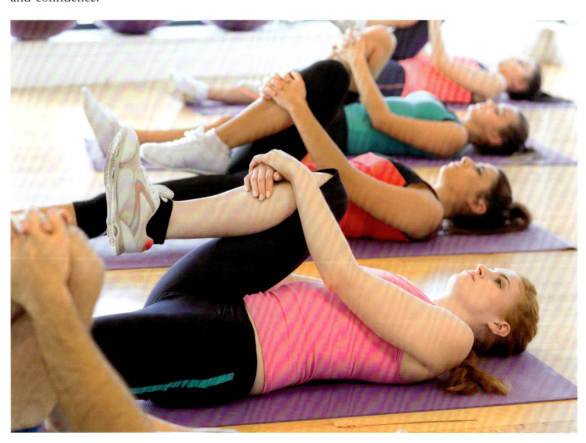

Figure 4.51 Legs up the wall pose, or Viparita Karani

(*Vee-pa-REE-tah Kah-rah-nee*, Sanskrit – Viparita Karani, Inverted or reversed position)

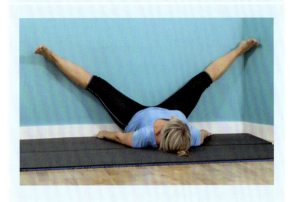

Purpose: A supine lying, inverted posture. Can be used as a progression towards inverted postures.

Benefits:
- Alleviates nervous exhaustion
- Improves circulation and venous return
- Reduces depression and boosts confidence
- Lengthens the hamstrings and adductors and erector spinae
- Relieves menstrual discomfort
- Relaxes the body
- Prevents varicose veins
- Relieves indigestion, diarrhoea and nausea
- Relieves breathlessness, asthma, palpitations and throat ailments

Suitable for: All levels

Precautions:
- Tightness in lower back or sciatica may prevent buttocks from touching wall: position buttocks further away
- Hip problems: perform without leg widening or with a smaller range of motion

Instructions and teaching points:
- Lie on one side in a foetal position with sitting bones against a wall
- Rotate to lie on the back with feet and buttocks against the wall
- Slide legs up the wall
- Relax the trunk
- Arms at a 45° angle away from body, palms face upwards
- Open the legs as wide as is comfortable
- Relax and breathe comfortably in the position

Progressions, modifications and variations:
- Knees can stay slightly bent
- Buttocks can be further away from wall
- Use pillow or cushion under lower back
- Extend legs, without taking legs apart
- Hands can provide support for outside of knees
- Straps can be used on each foot to assist leg widening (open and close)
- Progress to Upavistha Konasana
- Buttocks and lower back can be lifted higher by using a pillow to increase inversion

Visualisations:
- Root chakra connects to the wall
- Spine lengthens and opens, allowing energy to flow
- Tuck chin slightly inwards to connect throat chakra
- Crown chakra extends and opens away from body

Preparation: Knees bent and buttocks further away from wall

Counterpose: Knee-to-chest (Apanasana) or corpse

Figure 4.52 Corpse pose or Savasana
(*Shah-VAH-sa-na*, Sanskrit – Sava, Corpse)

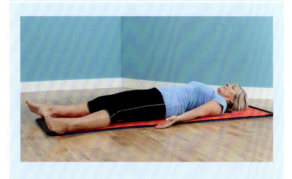

Purpose: A relaxation posture. Can be used as part of warm up and cool-down for relaxation components. A first step in practice of meditation

Benefits:
- Relaxes the whole body
- Allows the spine to rest, lengthen and relax
- Opens the hip joint
- Relaxes the shoulders and neck
- Releases physical and mental tension
- Calms the mind
- Helps to promote stillness to any inner turmoil or distress
- Improves venous return
- Optimal relaxation position for the spine, can assist realignment
- Lowers blood pressure
- Withdraws attention away from the senses
- Draws focus inwards towards the breath

Suitable for: All levels

Prohibitions: Pregnancy, trimesters 2 and 3

Precautions:
- Pregnancy: choose side lying position
- Lordosis: cushion or rolled up mat under lower back and possibly knees; or bend knees
- Knee hyperextension: block under knees
- Lower back problems: cushion under lower back or bend knees
- Kyphosis: block under head to prevent head tilting backwards

Instructions and teaching points:
- Lie supine on the back
- Feet hip width and a half apart
- Arms extended 5 inches away from side of body
- Palms face up and open fingers
- Shoulders relaxed and away from ears
- Neck lengthened
- Breathe comfortably
- Can practice abdominal breathing and full yogic breathing

Progressions, modifications and variations:
- Feet narrower
- Palms in comfortable position
- Side lying
- Knees bent and feet on floor – crook lying
- Legs on chair

Visualisations:
- Surrender and release body to the mat
- Surrender and release body and mind to the class
- Allow the mind to be here and now
- Allow the muscles to soften and relax
- Release and let go of all tension and tightness
- Allow the body and mind to become one with the breath
- Give permission to release and let go
- Allow withdrawal from the senses, which offer distraction

Preparation: Crook lying or can place cushion under knees

Counterpose: Knees-to-chest (Apanasana)

Figure 4.53 Wind-relieving pose, knees to chest pose or Apanasana

(*App-an-AAH-sa-na*, Sanskrit – Apana, waste eliminating)

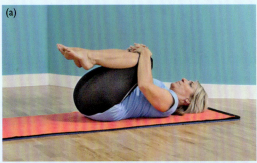
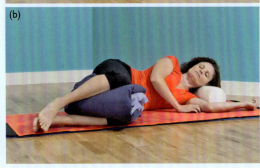

(a) Supine pose
(b) Side-lying pose

Purpose: A supine lying, resting pose. Can be used as a counterpose to strong spine extension postures (e.g. bridge, camel etc.)

Benefits:
- Relieves flatulence and constipation
- Stretches gluteals and erector spinae
- Lengthens spine
- Relieves tightness in hips and lower back
- Hip mobility
- Promotes sense of relaxation and calm

Suitable for: All levels

Precautions:
- Knee injury: hold back of thigh and smaller knee bend
- Pregnancy: left side lying option
- Round tummy: knees slightly apart

Instructions and teaching points:
- Lie supine on your back in corpse
- Bring legs together ankles touching
- On exhale bring one leg into the chest and then the other leg into the chest
- Hold the shins with the hands
- Relax the body into the floor
- Breathe comfortably

Progressions, modifications and variations:
- Hold the thighs rather than the shins
- Have the knees slightly apart
- Single leg variation (ardha apanasana)

Visualisations:
- Rock the back side to side or forwards and backwards to massage the spine
- Circle the knees gently clockwise and then anti-clockwise (visualising a pencil under the knees drawing a circle on the ceiling) to massage the lower back
- Feel the massaging effect on the abdominal region

Preparation: Half wind pose (single legs)

Counterpose: Corpse or full body stretch

Figure 4.54 Half wind-relieving pose or Ardha apanasana
(*Ard–hoo App-an-AAH-sa-na*, Sanskrit – Apana, waste eliminating)

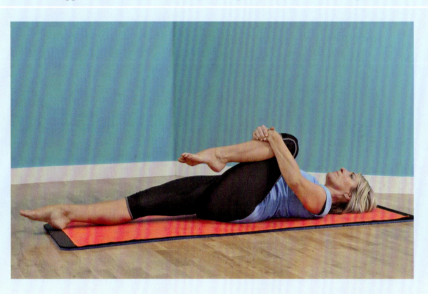

Purpose: A supine lying, resting pose. Can be used in warm up for mobility of hip

Benefits:
- Relieves flatulence and constipation
- Stretches gluteals and erector spinae (bent leg)
- Stretches hip flexor (straight leg)
- Lengthens spine
- Relieves tightness in hips and lower back
- Hip mobility and knee mobility (bent leg)
- Promotes sense of relaxation and calm

Suitable for: All levels

Precautions:
- Knee injury: hold back of thigh and smaller knee bend

Instructions and teaching points:
- From corpse position
- Exhale
- Bring one leg into the chest
- Hold the shins with the hands
- Inhale
- Return leg to the floor into corpse
- Repeat, with other leg

Progressions, modifications and variations:
- Hold the back of the thighs
- Hold the shins to increase range of motion slightly
- Have the knees slightly apart
- Hold for longer
- Both legs – Apanasana

Preparation: Smaller range of motion

Counterpose: Opposite side

Figure 4.55 Belly twist or Jathara Parivartanasana

(*Jath-Har-uh Par-ee-VAR-tahn-AAH-sa-na*, Sanskrit – Jathara, stomach; Parivartana, roll or turn around)

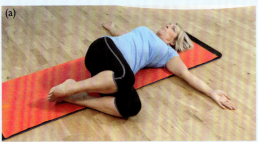

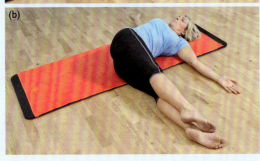

(a) Knees bent
(b) Progression with legs straight

Purpose: A twisting posture

Benefits:
- Mobility for spine and also knees and hips
- Stretches gluteals, erector spinae and obliques and pectoralis
- Opens the chest
- Relaxes the back
- Massages internal organs
- Improves digestion
- Wrings out any tension and frustration from the body
- Unblocks blocked energy in the spine

Suitable for: All levels

Precautions:
- Lower back pain: legs further away from buttocks
- Kyphosis or shoulder injury: palms can face upwards
- Kyphosis: may need block to support head and prevent backward tilt, blocks under knees and smaller rotation

Instructions and teaching points:
- From Corpse
- Bend knees with feet on floor and heels against buttocks
- Arms in crucifix position, level with chest – palms face down
- Inhale and engage abdominals
- Exhale
- Rotate to one side
- Lower knees slowly towards the floor (aiming towards a 90° rotation)
- Keep feet and knees together
- Rotate head to look to opposite side
- Keep shoulder blades on the floor
- Breathe naturally
- Relax into position
- Repeat on other side

Progressions, modifications and variations:
- Palms can face upwards
- Smaller rotation – 45°
- Legs can be further away from buttocks
- Can progress to straightening legs once rotated

Visualisations:
- Wringing out tension from the spine
- Release and let go of any blocks to energy

Preparation: Smaller range of motion

Counterpose: Opposite side and knee-to-chest (Apanasana)

Figure 4.56 Reclined Cobbler's pose or Supta Baddhakonasana
(*Soopta Bhaad-dah-kohn-AAH-sa-na*, Sanskrit – Baddha, bound or caught; Kona, angle)

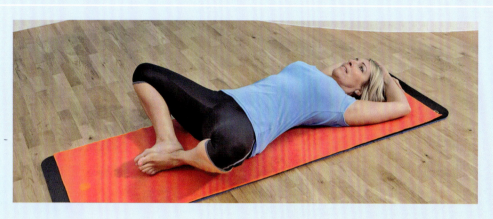

Image shows progression

Purpose: A relaxation posture to open the hips

Benefits:
- Stretches adductors
- Promotes relaxation
- Opens the hips
- Hip and knee mobility
- Helps to relieve sacroiliac pain and discomfort
- Reduces sciatic pain
- Conserves energy

Suitable for: All levels

Prohibitions: Pregnancy

Precautions:
- Tight hips or knee ligament problems: blocks under knees

Instructions and teaching points:
- From corpse
- Bend the knees to crook position with feet on floor
- Allow the hips to open, so that knees move towards the floor, soles of feet together
- Lengthen spine and neck
- Hands at a 45° angle from body and palms face upwards
- Breathe comfortably to hold position

Progressions, modifications and variations:
- Seated version
- Legs further away
- Legs closer
- Progress to Viparita Karani or Legs up the wall pose or Inverted lake pose
- Lower back can be supported with cushion
- Blocks under knees
- Hands behind the crown of the head, as pictured

Visualisations:
- Relax back and take a breath, surrender to the opening of the hips

Preparation: Corpse pose (Savasana)

Counterpose: Knees-to-chest (Apanasana)

Figure 4.57 Child's pose or Balasana
(*Bahl-AAH-sa-na*, Sanskrit – Bala, child)

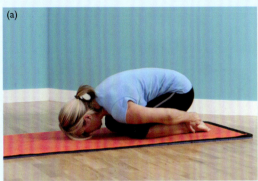

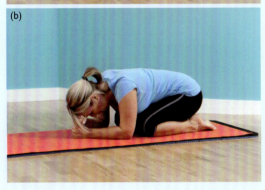

(a) Full position holding ankles
(b) Modification – hands under forehead

Purpose: A resting and flexed posture. Can be used as a counterpose to strong spine extension postures

Benefits:
- Lengthens gluteals and erector spinae and tibalis anterior
- Stretches ankles
- Releases tension on lower back
- Stimulates digestion
- Restores a sense of calm and positive energy
- Releases frustration

Precautions:
- Kyphosis: place head on block or double fist
- Knee problems or lower back: pillow under heels
- Round shoulders: can place blocks under shoulders or engage lower trapezius to draw shoulder blades towards buttocks

Instructions and teaching points:
- Kneel on the floor, buttocks resting on heels
- Connect with the solar plexus
- Bend forward from hips and rest chest on thighs
- Place forehead on floor or on a block
- Spine lengthens
- Arms at side of body, close to ankles
- Palms face upwards
- Extend fingers
- Open and lengthen the spine

Progressions, modifications and variations:
- Block or pillow between buttocks and heels
- Knees open slightly
- Block under forehead
- Hands under forehead, either flat or double fist to elevate head
- Arms can extend in front
- Hands hold ankles

Visualisations:
- Third eye chakra connects with floor
- Chin tucks inwards to connect throat chakra
- Solar plexus and heart chakras connect with thighs
- Surrender to the posture
- Upper body surrenders to lower body

Preparation: Smaller range of motion with buttocks lifted slightly

Counterpose: Cow (see mobility sequence)

INVERTED POSTURES – INVERSIONS

Inversions or inverted postures are the 'upside down' postures, where the head is lower than the heart. Inversions have benefits for the lymphatic, circulatory, nervous and endocrine systems. The inverted position increases blood flow to the endocrine glands in the upper regions of the body, giving them a flush of oxygenated blood and a recharge that helps to boost the immune system and hormonal balance.

When inverted, gravity assists with tissue drainage from the lower body by reversing the regular flow of blood and lymph. The inverted postures will also strengthen the muscles of the upper body that assist with holding the positions.

Psychologically, the inversions can instil feelings of confidence, calm and tranquillity, not least, because they demand great focus and attention.

The *Hatha Yoga Pradipika* describes the head stand and shoulder stand, respectively, as the 'king' and 'queen' of postures because they enhance the health of body and mind.

Figure 4.58 Downward-facing dog, or Adho Mukha Shvanasana
(*Ad-ho Muuk-ha-shvan-HAA-sa-na*, Sanskrit – Adho, downwards; Mukha, face; Shvana, dog)

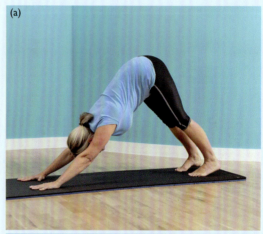

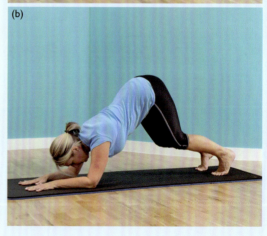

(a) Full position
(b) Modification, half downwards dog

Purpose: An inverted posture. It can be used as a preparatory mobility posture. One posture within the sun salutation – Surya Namaskara

Benefits:
- Strengthens medial deltoids, biceps and triceps (to lift and hold position)
- Stretches hamstrings, gluteals, erector spinae, gastrocnemius, latissimus dorsi, pectorals and anterior deltoid
- Strengthens abdominal and shoulder girdle stabilisers
- Mobilises hip, knee, shoulder, elbow and ankle
- Stimulates diaphragm and heart
- Assists venous return
- Increase blood flow to brain (Inversion)

Suitable for: All levels

Prohibitions:
- Carpal tunnel syndrome or RSI of wrist
- High blood pressure
- Glaucoma or other eye problems
- Recurrent shoulder dislocation

Precautions:
- Tight hamstrings or lower back: bend knees
- Knee hyperextension: keep knees unlocked
- Pregnancy: after first trimester use Cat pose
- Wrist problems: rest hands in fist position to align wrist
- As part of preparatory phase: perform modifications first, to build range of motion

Instructions and teaching points:
- From all fours, with hands under shoulders and fingers spread
- Middle finger points forward
- Knees under hips and feet at hip width
- Inhale
- Plant feet or balls of the foot on the floor
- Exhale
- Push through the hands and lift buttocks towards the ceiling, straightening legs
- Knees and elbows unlocked
- Create an inverted 'V' shape
- Ease the chest towards the knees and heels towards the floor
- Neck in line with eyes focused towards the tips of the toes
- Shoulder blades slide down towards buttocks
- Arm pits rotate inwards
- Breathe comfortably to hold position
- Lower on an inhalation

Progressions, modifications and variations:
- Half downward dog with knees bent
- Child's pose
- Blocks under hands
- Blocks under heels
- Hands on a step to reduce range of motion
- Use fists instead of spread hands (option to use press up bars, if available to align wrists)
- Heels lifted
- Progress by easing chest closer to thighs and heels closer to floor

Visualisations:
- Root chakra lifts to ceiling
- Crown chakra extends to floor
- Release tension in lower back

Preparation: Modified version with bent knees; child's pose or elevated child's pose

Counterpose: Cow (from Cat to Cow sequence) or other gentle back bend

Figure 4.59 Half shoulder stand or Ardha Sarvangasana

(*Ahr-dha Sahr-vaang-AAH-sa-na*, Sanskrit – Ardha, half; Sarva, all; anga, limb)

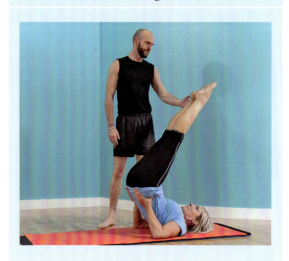

Purpose: An inverted and balancing posture

Benefits:
- Strengthens abdominals and core spine stabilisers
- Strengthens quadriceps, gluteals, hamstrings, adductors to hold position
- Assists venous return
- Relieves blood pooling from lower limbs
- Increase circulation of blood to the brain
- Stimulates the thyroid gland (throat chakra)
- Helps prevent varicose veins
- Helps to relieve insomnia

Suitable for: Intermediate/Advanced

Prohibitions:
- Cardiac conditions
- High blood pressure
- Eye or ear problems
- Osteoporosis
- Hernia
- Neck or shoulder injuries
- Kyphosis

Precautions:
- Use modifications for any neck issues, hypertension, glaucoma, wrist or elbow issues, menstruation

Instructions and teaching points:
- Lie supine on back with knees bent and heels to buttocks
- Place hands underneath the buttocks as if reaching for feet
- Bring elbows as close together as possible
- Push through hands and roll knees to chest, lifting buttocks and lower back away from the floor
- Inhale
- Hands support lower back, elbows on floor
- Exhale
- Engage abdominals
- Extend legs to ceiling, keeping legs together, knees slightly bent
- Body weight on shoulders and arms (NOT the neck)
- Chest to chin
- Focus on the throat
- Breathe comfortably to hold position

Progressions, modifications and variations:
- Bridge is modification
- Pillow or pad under neck and shoulder area
- Perform close to wall and feet on wall to assist balance

Visualisations:
- Focus on throat chakra

Preparation: Half shoulder stand

Counterpose: Cobra, Sphinx or Corpse

Figure 4.60 Shoulder stand or Sarvangasana

(*Sahr-vaang-AAH-sa-na*, Sanskrit – Sarva, all; anga, limb)

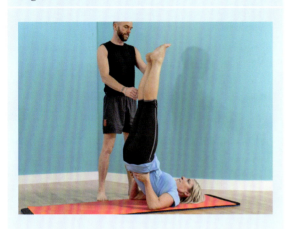

Purpose: An inverted and balancing posture

Benefits:
- Strengthens abdominals and core spine stabilisers
- Strengthens quadriceps, gluteals, hamstrings, adductors to hold position
- Assists venous return
- Relieves blood pooling from lower limbs
- Increases circulation of blood to the brain
- Stimulates the thyroid gland (throat chakra)
- Helps prevent varicose veins
- Helps to relieve insomnia

Suitable for: Advanced

Prohibitions:
- Cardiac conditions
- High blood pressure
- Eye or ear problems
- Osteoporosis
- Hernia
- Neck or shoulder injuries
- Kyphosis

Precautions:
- Use modifications for any neck issues, hypertension, glaucoma, wrist or elbow issues, menstruation

Instructions and teaching points:
- Lie supine on back with knees bent and heels to buttocks
- Place hands underneath the buttocks as if reaching for feet
- Bring elbows as close together as possible
- Push through hands and roll knees to chest, lifting buttocks and lower back away from the floor
- Inhale
- Hands support lower back, elbows on floor
- Exhale
- Engage abdominals
- Extend legs to ceiling, keeping legs together, legs straight
- Walk the hands down towards shoulder blades to lift higher
- Body weight on shoulders and arms (NOT the neck)
- Chest to chin
- Breathe comfortably to hold position

Progressions, modifications and variations:
- Bridge is modification
- Half shoulder stand
- Pillow or pad under neck and shoulder area
- Perform close to wall and feet on wall to assist balance

Visualisations:
- Focus on third eye chakra (between eyebrows) to increase focus and relaxation
- Throat chakra stimulated by breath

Preparation: Single/Double leg raise, Viparita Kirani, Ardha Sarvangasana (half shoulder stand)

Counterpose: Half or full fish

Figure 4.61 Plough or Halasana
(*Hal-AAH-sa-na*, Sanskrit – Hala, plough)

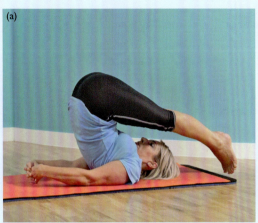

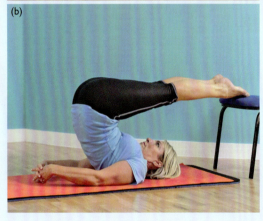

(a) Full position
(b) Modification – feet on a chair to decrease ROM

Purpose: An inverted and balancing posture. Flexes and stretches the spine

Benefits:
- Stretches erector spinae, gluteals, hamstrings, gastrocnemius and upper trapezius (back of neck)
- Mobilises spine and hips
- Stimulates the thyroid gland (throat chakra)
- Stimulates abdominal organs and digestion

Suitable for: Advanced

Prohibitions:
- Back or neck injuries
- High blood pressure
- Vertigo
- Glaucoma
- Cardiac or respiratory conditions

Precautions:
- Use modifications for any neck, spine or hip issues, hypertension, glaucoma, claustrophobia issues

Instructions and teaching points:
- From shoulder stand with hands supporting lower back
- Lower right leg to floor behind head
- Lower left leg to floor behind head
- Both feet touching floor
- Extend arms to floor (can clasp hands and press into floor)

Progressions, modifications and variations:
- Modification: apanasana, with or without small lift of body, supported with hands
- Feet on a block or a chair instead of floor
- Hands remain supporting back

Visualisations:
- Your body makes the shape of a horse-drawn plough

Preparation: Apanasana and half shoulder stand

Counterpose: Bridge or Corpse

Figure 4.62 Crane pose, Crow pose, or Bakasana

(*Bak-AAH-sa-na*, Sanskrit – Baka, crane, heron)

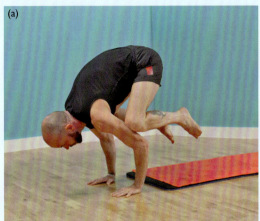

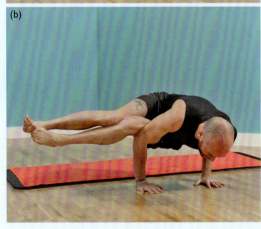

(a) Crane pose
(b) Progression crow pose twisted

Purpose: A balancing and strengthening posture

Benefits:
- Strengthens triceps, biceps, deltoids, upper and middle trapezius, rhomboids
- Strengthens wrists and forearms
- Strengthens core abdominal muscles to hold position
- Assists balance
- Lengthens gluteals and erector spinae

Suitable for: Intermediate and Advanced

Prohibitions:
- Carpal tunnel syndrome
- Pregnancy

Precautions
- Wrist or elbow issues, weak core, balance issues

Instructions and teaching points:
- From Garland position or Hindi squat
- Elbows into knees
- Take hands forward, spread fingers and turn hands slightly inwards
- Elbows bent
- Lift up on to balls of feet, taking weight slightly forward
- Bring thighs towards chest and shins towards upper arms
- Slowly lift feet to find balance point, keep head aligned
- Breathe comfortably to hold position

Progressions, modifications and variations:
- Garland
- Forward lean with full balance
- Raised cushions under forehead to reduce fears of losing balance
- Twisted variation from twisted chair and balancing both legs on to one arm (Parsva bakasana) see image (b) opposite.

Visualisations:
- Focus on a point on the floor

Preparation: Hindi squat or garland

Counterpose: Sitting straight-legged with arms above head pose (Utthita Hasta Dandasana)

Figure 4.63 Head stand or Sirsasana
(*Sheer-SAAH-sa-na*, Sanskrit – Shirsa, head)

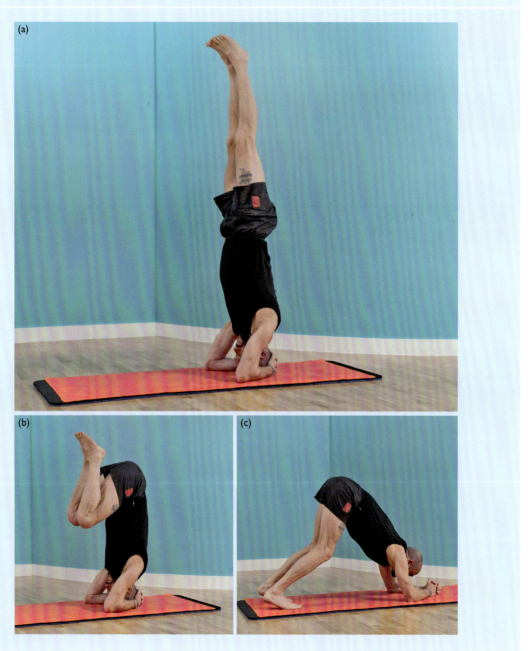

(a) Full head stand
(b) Half head stand
(c) Dolphin

Purpose: A fully inverted and balancing posture

Benefits:
- Strengthens abdominals and core spine stabilisers
- Strengthens quadriceps, gluteals, hamstrings, adductors, deltoids, triceps, biceps to hold position
- Assists venous return
- Relieves blood pooling from lower limbs
- Increased circulation of blood to the brain
- Stimulates the thyroid gland (throat chakra)
- Helps prevent varicose veins
- Helps to relieve insomnia
- Improves self confidence

Suitable for: Advanced

Prohibitions:
- Cardiac conditions
- High blood pressure
- Eye or ear problems
- Osteoporosis
- Hernia
- Neck or shoulder injuries
- Kyphosis
- Pregnancy
- Obesity
- Heavy cold

Precautions:
- Use modification for any minor neck or head issues, hypertension, balance issues, beginners, menstruation

Instructions and teaching points:
- From child's pose
- Come to all fours and bend elbows so forearms rest on floor, hands are able to touch opposite elbow
- Clasp hands and move them forward, under forehead, forming a triangle shape
- Shoulders away from ears and lengthen the neck
- Bring crown of head to floor with back of head supported in hands
- Push up on to toes, straightening the legs
- Walk the feet in towards the head, sitting bones high, until spine is as straight as possible
- Balance weight through elbows and hands, gentle pressure on crown
- Gently lift one leg bending at knee
- Once balanced gently lift other leg, keeping knee bent *(dolphin pose achieved)*
- Raise legs so that knees are in line with spine, knees still bent
- When balanced float feet up, legs straight
- Keeping shoulders away from ears
- Breathe comfortably to hold position

Progressions, modifications and variations:
- Bridge
- Downward dog
- Dolphin with knees bent
- Use a wall for balance
- Partner can support legs

Visualisations:
- Turn your world upside down

Preparation: Downward dog or dolphin with child's pose before taking the pose

Counterpose: Shoulder stand to ease pressure on the neck and child's pose (Balasana) to release tension from the back

PRANAYAMA – BREATH WORK/REGULATION AND CONTROL

When the breath is unsteady, the mind is unsteady. When the breath is steady, the mind is steady and the yogi becomes steady. Therefore one should restrain the breath.
   Hatha Yoga Pradipika, Svatmarama, Ch 2 vs 1, 2

WHAT IS PRANAYAMA?

Pranayama (pronounced Prah-naah-YAHM-ah) is the fourth limb of yoga (Yoga Sutras). It is an essential component of yoga practice because the breath is an 'extension of the life force' and pranic energy.

The word pranayama evolves from Sanskrit language and is formed by two words – prana and ayama.
- Prana means the 'life force', the breath, the internal energy (Pra – before, and An – to breathe or to live)
- Ayama means control, extension.

Pranayama practice offers a way to extend the life force and/or control the breath. The Yoga Sutras (2.49) describe pranayama as the interruption of the inward and outward flow of the breath (Swami Satchidanada, 1990) (see Kumbaka, discussed later).

WHY PRACTICE PRANAYAMA?

There are many benefits for practising breath work and pranayama, these include:
- Psychological benefits
- Physiological benefits
- Energetic benefits.

PSYCHOLOGICAL BENEFITS

Focusing on the breath during asana practice, and also during relaxation and meditation practice, restores mental clarity and connects the mind and body, creating a shared or joined consciousness or connectedness.

Breath work provides a focus that can help to reduce the inner chatter of the mind and helps to provide a release from stress and enables a connection with the higher, spiritual self.

Breath work also helps to improve emotional and physical control, promotes inner balance and tranquillity and raises awareness of the different rhythms of the body.

Pranayama fits the mind for meditation. It can be used for purification.
   The Yoga Sutras, 2.53 (Swami Satchidanada, 1990)

PHYSIOLOGICAL BENEFITS
Breath work delivers oxygenated blood to the working muscles and cells of the body; it also assists with removal of waste (carbon dioxide). It cleanses the airways and some practices can be useful in the management of respiratory conditions.

ENERGETIC BENEFITS
Prana is energy, so by focusing on the breath, the life force is positively encouraged to move through the different energy channels or nadis of the energy body.

> *Pranayama removes obstruction to enlightenment.*
> The Yoga Sutras, 2.52, (Swami Satchidanada, 1990)

> *The breath splits open the mouth of the Sushumna and enters easily once all the nadis are purified by restraining prana correctly.*
> *Hatha Yoga Pradipika*, Svatmarama, Ch 2 vs 41

HOW TO PRACTICE BREATH WORK AND PRANAYAMA?
There are many different breathing exercises, from simple and basic techniques, to more advanced techniques. Many of the more advanced techniques should only be practised under the supervision and guidance of an experienced teacher.

NASAL BREATHING
Nasal breathing, or breathing in and out through the nose, allows for a fuller and deeper breath. It helps to filter and warm the air. It can also provide the focus needed for practice by bringing the individual's attention to the here and now, which is the essence of yoga practice: being present and mindful.

This method is the most commonly practised when performing asana. See full abdominal breathing and yogic breath instructions (page 153).

MOUTH BREATHING
Mouth breathing, is often a cooler breathing action and usually shallower. This is because the nostrils are very narrow so once inhaled, the air heats up through the passage to the throat. Breathing through a wide mouth allows much more air to rush in and is a much larger space. This sudden influx of air hits the back of the throat and is much cooler. Some of the advanced breathing methods use mouth breathing (see sithali breathing instructions, page 157).

SAMAVRTTI OR SAME ACTION BREATHING
Breathing patterns are often irregular and shallow. Focusing on the irregularities of the breath and allowing the breath to become slower and more even will calm the mind and create a feeling of balance and stability. Inhaling for four counts and exhaling for four counts will help to develop Samavrtti or same action breathing.

As a starter practice, focus awareness to the four stages of the breath:
- Stage 1: Inhale
- Stage 2: Slight pause
- Stage 3: Exhale
- Stage 4: Slight pause

Beginners should just focus on breathing rhythmically and evenly and will often use shorter breathing ratios, for example: inhale for four counts, exhale for four counts with only a slight pause and no retention.

Advanced practitioners can use retention (see kumbaka) during the pause phases at the end of the inhale and exhale stages.

The stages of the breath can be introduced during the initial relaxation at the start of practice and the flow of breath can be maintained during asana practice.

UJJAYI BREATHING OR VICTORIOUS BREATH

Ujjayi breathing can be developed from Samavrtti or same action breathing. The same breathing rhythm is maintained, but the mouth is closed and the epiglottis is constricted (like breathing though a hole in the throat), creating a 'throaty' or hissing sound. Ujjayi is sometimes known as 'ocean breath' because the inner sound is much like that of the tides of the ocean as they flow.

Ujjayi breathing improves concentration, calms the body and mind and soothes the nervous system. It is used in yoga therapy for this reason. Ujjayi also tones the internal organs and increases inner temperature, generating heat and is most often used in Ashtanga yoga practices. It is not recommended for individuals with a hot temperament or those who are introverted to do this without supervision, as they may not be used to such energy rushes that stimulate the sympathetic system.

KUMBAKA BREATHING OR BREATH RETENTION

Kumbaka breathing is the practice of breath retention or holding the breath. It is a more advanced technique. It cleanses the respiratory system and strengthens the diaphragm, restoring energy.

Some believe that we are born with a set number of breaths during incarnation and by learning to slow the breathing, we can achieve Samadhi before the final breath occurs. Life is determined by breath and having the desire to free oneself from the cycle of birth and death. The practice of breath allows the yogi to attain 'moksha' or liberation.

Kumbaka practice:
- **Purak**: inhalation
- **Rechak**: exhalation
- **Kumbak**: retention of breath
- **Antar kumbak**: internal retention (Antar – retain energy). Hold breath for longer after inhalation
- **Bahir kumbak**: external retention (Bahir – retain breath outside of the body). Hold breath for longer after exhalation. *NB: This is an advanced practice, as breath retention outside is believed to be as close to death as one can get.*

Kumbaka can initially be practised at the end of the session, during the closing phase of practice and while in a seated meditation position.
- When starting, four natural rhythm breaths can be taken and after each fourth inhale, the breath can be held in, initially for around four to eight counts. To progress from this:
- The exhale can start with the same number of counts as the inhale (e.g. four counts) but can steadily be increased over time.

Table 5.1	Breathing ration guidelines			
Level	Inhale	Retention	Exhale	Retention
Absolute beginners	1 inhale (4 counts)	No retention	1 exhale (4 counts)	No retention
Beginners	1 inhale (4 counts)	1 retention (4 counts)	1 exhale (4 counts)	No retention
Intermediate	1 inhale (4 counts)	2 retention (8 counts)	2 exhale (8 counts)	No retention

- The number of breaths between kumbaka practice can reduce, so that it is practised during every breath cycle
- The number of counts during Purak, Rechak and Kumbak can be increased over time.

PRECAUTIONS AND PROHIBITIONS FOR PRANAYAMA PRACTICE

The following should all be taken into account prior to practising pranyama.

- Practice on an empty stomach, ideally four hours after eating a meal
- Maintain flow and avoid forcing or straining the breath
- Feelings of dizziness or feeling unwell: stop practice
- Colds or respiratory problems: defer practice
- Pregnancy: avoid pumping breath or breath retention
- High blood pressure: avoid breath retention
- High blood pressure, heart disease or vertigo: avoid Bhastrika or Kapalabhati
- Cold individuals: avoid sitali and sitkari (cold practices)
- Hot individuals: avoid ujjayi (hot practices).

Precautions for other specific practices are discussed under the instructions for each practice.

Figure 5.1 Deep abdominal breathing: corpse pose

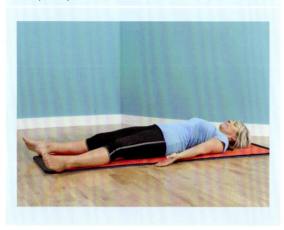

The hands can be placed on the tummy, with the tip of the middle fingers touching at the belly button. During inhalation, the fingertips will move apart. During exhalation, the fingertips will move back together.

Purpose: This is the simplest method of breathing. It brings focus to breathing patterns, which are often shallow (usually upper chest breathing)

Benefits:
- Brings attention to the breath
- Focuses the mind
- Promotes relaxation

Suitable for: All levels

Instructions and teaching points:
- In a comfortable relaxation position (e.g. Corpse)
- Bring the awareness to the breath
- Inhale through the nose slowly and deeply
- Allow the abdominals (belly button) to rise on the inhale
- Ribs and chest are relaxed
- Exhale through the nose slowly and deeply
- Allow the abdominals to fall, the belly deflates

Modifications and variations:
- Corpse or other lying positions
- Virasana (Hero)
- Sukhasana (Cross-legged) or other seated postures
- Foetus position (side lying)
- Any position that feels comfortable and promotes relaxation

Visualisation:
- Exhale anger, frustration, fatigue and disease
- Inhale love, light, relaxation, energy and health

Figure 5.2 Full yogic breath

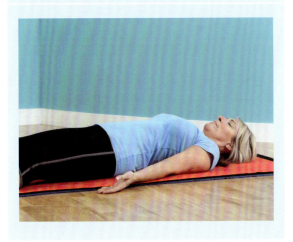

> Some schools of yoga will inhale and expand the upper chest first (chest, ribs, abdomen) and exhale in reverse (abdomen, ribs, chest). It is believed that this pattern stretches the spine and the back more fully, (Desikachar, 1999:22)

Purpose: This is a progression from abdominal breathing and can be taught at the beginning of a session and used while performing all asanas. It is a progression towards ujjayi breathing.

Benefits:
- Brings attention to the breath
- Focuses the mind
- Promotes relaxation of the chest, back and shoulders
- Inflates the lungs more fully

Suitable for: All levels

Instructions and teaching points:
- In a comfortable relaxation position (e.g. Corpse)
- Bring the awareness to the breath
- Inhale through the nose slowly and deeply
  - Allow the abdominals (belly button) to rise on the inhale
  - Ribs expand laterally
  - Collarbone and sternum rise
- Exhale through the nose slowly and deeply
  - Allow the abdominals to fall, the belly deflates
  - Ribcage relaxes
  - Collarbone and chest relax
- Air pushes gently, not forcefully from the lungs

Modifications and variations:
- Corpse or other lying positions
- Virasana (hero)
- Sukhasana (cross-legged) or other seated postures
- Foetus position (side lying)
- Any position that feels comfortable and promotes relaxation

Visualisation:
- Exhale anger, frustration, fatigue and disease
- Inhale love, light, relaxation, energy and health

Figure 5.3 Hummingbee or Brahmari breath

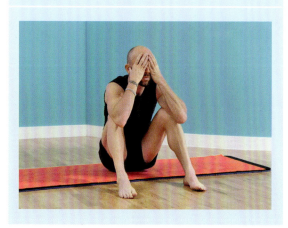

Purpose: Brahmari breath is a deep and restorative practice which can relieve anxiety and anger and promote a sense of calm and improved emotional well-being. Brahmari offers a way of listening inwardly to the breath, which helps to reconnect with the inner rhythms.

Benefits:
- Brings attention to the inner sound and rhythm of the breath
- Increases a sense of well-being
- Relieves anxiety and stress
- Reduces anger
- Can help to lower blood pressure
- Assists with healing
- Eliminates throat problems

Suitable for: All levels

Instructions and teaching points:
- Sit in a comfortable seated position (lying positions are NOT appropriate)
- Spine lengthened and shoulders relaxed away from the ears
- Thumbs press gently to close the ears, to close out other auditory noise
- Fingers gently over the eyes to close off the visual senses
- Mouth closed, teeth slightly apart
- Inhale through the nose
- Exhale and create a humming sound (like a bumblebee) at the back of the throat
- Body remains still
- Shoulders relaxed
- Repeat up to five times using a comfortable breathing ratio

Start position: Modifications and variations:
- Sukhasana (cross-legged) or other seated postures
- Seated with feet on the floor and knees bent, arms resting on knees

Visualisation:
- Exhale anger, frustration, fatigue and disease
- Inhale love, light, relaxation, energy and health

A quick and resonant inhalation sounding like a bee; a very slow exhalation sounding like a female bee. Thus a certain bliss and delight are born in the minds of good yogis from doing Brahmari.

Hatha Yoga Pradipika, Svatmarama, Chapter 2. vs 68

Figure 5.4 Alternate nostril breathing – Nadi Sodhana

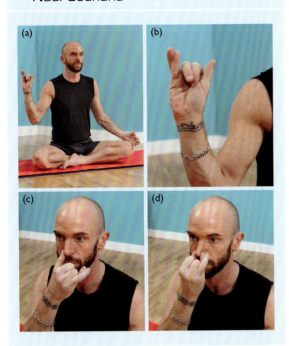

Translation: Nadi means channel; Sodhana means purification

Purpose: Purifies the energy channels by supplying oxygen to the body, inducing a sense of tranquility

Benefits:
- Brings in increased oxygen for the body
- Cleanses and purifies the energy channels or nadis
- Reduces stress and anxiety
- Promotes clarity of thought
- Increases concentration and focus
- Enhances a sense of tranquillity
- Balances ida and pingala, enabling Sushumna nadi to flow
- Assists with meditation and spiritual awakening

Suitable for: Intermediate. Supervision recommended. Ujjayi breathing NOT to be used with nostril breathing.

Instructions and teaching points:
- Sit in Sukhasana, or a comfortable seated posture
- Spine long
- Left hand in chin mudra (see page 164), resting above left knee
- Right hand in Vishnu mudra (see page 164)
- Shoulder relaxed and down, arm relaxed
  - Place right thumb next to right nostril and close the nostril with the thumb
  - Exhale through the left nostril for four counts (Om 1, Om 2, Om 3, Om 4)
  - Inhale through the left nostril for four counts (Om 1, Om 2, Om 3, Om 4)
  - Close off the left nostril with the ring finger and little finger
  - Open the right nostril by removing the right thumb away from nostril
  - Exhale through the right nostril for four counts (Om 1, Om 2, Om 3, Om 4)
  - Inhale through the right nostril for four counts (Om 1, Om 2, Om 3, Om 4)
  - One breathing round is complete
- Repeat up to 12 rounds, ratio can be varied

Modifications and variations:
- Sukhasana, Siddhasana or half or full lotus
- Seated, with a block or blanket under buttocks, to increase comfort
- Seated, with blocks or blankets under knees, to increase comfort
- Reduce the length of the breath count to increase comfort
- Other variations include inhaling through both nostrils and exhaling through alternate nostrils and vice versa

Figure 5.5 Lung-cleansing exercise – Kapalabhati

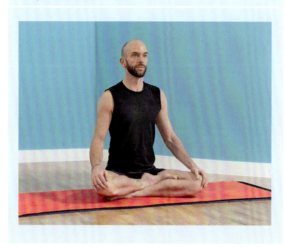

Purpose: Kapalabhati is a lung-cleansing pranayama exercise and is also one of the six Kriyas or purifying techniques used by Yogis. It is sometimes known as 'shiny skull'.

Benefits:
- Pushes stale air from the lungs enabling more space for fresh air and oxygen to enter

Suitable for: Advanced and experiencd only! Supervision recommended.

Prohibitions:
- Pregnancy
- Individuals with high blood pressure, sinus or ear blockages, glaucoma

Instructions and teaching points:
Part 1:
- In a comfortable seated position – Sukhasana (cross-legged) or half/full lotus
- Lengthen through spine
- Take two full yogic breaths and exhale completely
- Inhale
- Exhale and pull in abdomen (rest of body remains still)
- Inhale, relax the abdomen
- Maintain rhythmic breathing action
- Emphasise the exhalation
- 20 pumps for the first round

Part 2:
- Take two full yogic breaths and exhale completely
- Inhale and retain the breath for around 30 seconds
- Maintain comfortable and upright seated posture
- Body is still
- Can repeat (see modifications and variations)

Modifications and variations:
- Virasana (hero) or other seated postures
- Use a mat under sitting bones
- Can repeat up to 3 times
- Can increase pumps to 20, 40 or 60
- Can increase retention to 30–40 or 60 seconds

Visualisation:
- During pumping, the teacher cues '1, **2**, 1, **2**, 1, **2**, 1, **2**', emphasising the 2 as the outward breath

Figure 5.6 Cooling breath – Sithali

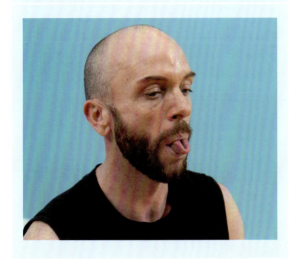

Purpose: A cooling breath to promote physical and mental tranquillity. Sithali is the Sanskrit word for sheet and means 'cool'.

Benefits:
- Helps to cool the body and mind
- Promotes mental and physical tranquility
- Helps to control hunger and thirst
- Reduces blood pressure and acid stomach

Suitable for: Advanced. Supervision recommended.

Prohibitions:
- Low blood pressure (avoid the technique)
- Asthma and respiratory conditions
- Excess mucus

Precautions:
- Pregnancy (no breath retention)
- High blood pressure (no breath retention)
- Avoid practice in cold climates or seasons

Instructions and teaching points:
- In a comfortable seated position – Sukhasana (cross-legged) or half/full lotus
- Lengthen through spine
- Hands in chin mudra (see page 164)
- Stick the tongue out a little and curl the sides of the tongue up and inwards to make a straw or tube shape; through which to sip the air
- Inhale slowly and gently through the mouth, with tongue in tube shape
- Close the mouth and retain breath for as long as is comfortable
- Exhale gently through the nose, keeping the mouth closed
- This is one round
- 5 to 10 rounds can be performed

Modifications and variations:
- Virasana (Hero) or other seated postures
- Use a mat under sitting bones
- More advanced can activate jalandhara (see page 166) and moola bandha (see page 168) during retention
- Increase rounds up to 10

Figure 5.7 Cooling or hissing breath – Sitkari

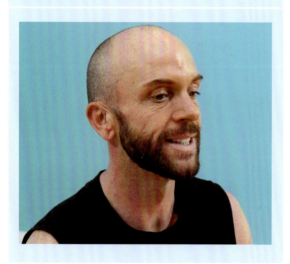

Purpose: A cooling breath to promote clarity of thought, concentration and physical and mental tranquillity. Offers the same benefits of Sithali breath, as well as keeping teeth and gums healthy

Benefits:
- Brings extra oxygen to the body
- Helps to cool the body and mind
- Reduces stress and anxiety
- Brings clarity of thought and concentration
- Promotes mental and physical tranquillity
- Balances ida and pingala, causing Sushumna nadi to flow, assisting with meditation and spiritual awakening
- Helps to control hunger and thirst
- Reduces blood pressure and acid stomach

Suitable for: Advanced. Supervision recommended.

Prohibitions: It is not recommended for practice by persons of a cold disposition

Precautions:
- If uncomfortable, reduce the breath count
- Sensitive teeth, practise Sithali

Instructions and teaching points:
- In a comfortable seated position – Sukhasana (cross-legged) or half/full lotus
- Lengthen through spine
- Hands in chin mudra (see page 164)
- Open the mouth
- Teeth gently together
- Place tongue behind the upper teeth with the tip of the tongue pressing on the palate
- Inhale slowly through the mouth making a hissing sound
- Close the mouth
- Exhale slowly through the nose
- This is one round, can repeat up to nine rounds

Modifications and variations:
- Virasana (hero) or other seated postures
- Use a mat under sitting bones
- Increase rounds up to nine

Figure 5.8 Vitality stimulating breath – Surya Bhedana

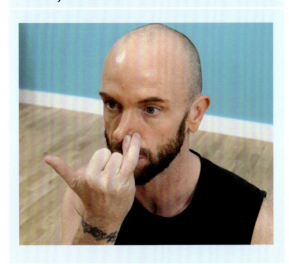

Purpose: Surya Bhedana is an excellent pre-meditation pranayama. It creates heat and activates pingala nadi, stimulating and awakening pranic energy. Surya is Sanskrit for 'sun' (referring to pingala nadi) and bheda is Sanskrit for 'pierce'

Benefits:
- Creates heat in the body
- Stimulates the mind and makes it more alert
- Helps to increase energy
- Can help to alleviate depression and low mood
- Activates pingala nadi and stimulates pranic energy

Suitable for: Advanced, and only under supervision

Prohibitions: It is not recommended for practice by persons of a cold disposition

Precautions:
- Not to be practised after eating
- Practise for no longer than 30 minutes

Instructions and teaching points:
- Seated in Sukhasana or other meditation posture, body relaxed
- Hands in chin mudra
- Focus on the nostrils
- Right hand into Vishnu mudra
- Close the left nostril with right ring finger
- Inhale slowly and deeply through right nostril
- Close both nostrils
- Activate jalandhara and moola bandhas
- Hold for a few seconds
- Release the bandhas
- When head is upright, exhale slowly through right nostril
- Keep the left nostril closed with the ring finger of right hand
- This is one round

Modifications and variations:
- Virasana (Hero) or other seated meditation postures
- Use a mat under sitting bones
- Can use a block under knees
- New to practice: 10 rounds and 10–15 minutes maximum
- Breath ratio of 1:1: 1:0, increasing to 1:2: 2:0

Figure 5.9 Bellows breathing – Bhastrika

Purpose: Bhastrika or bellows breathing fans the flame of gastric fire by drawing air forcibly into and out of the lungs

Benefits:
- Generates heat
- Burns off apana (waste accumulated) in the abdominal region

Suitable for: Advanced. Supervision recommended.

Prohibitions:
- High blood pressure
- Heart disease
- Glaucoma
- Pregnancy

Precautions:
- Not to be practised after eating
- Stop if dizziness experienced
- Stop if nose bleeds
- Take three months to build up to three rounds of twenty pumps

Instructions and teaching points:
- Blow the nose or practise neti (see page 170) before practising
- In a comfortable meditation position, e.g. Sukhasana
- Inhale in a quick burst, expanding abdomen
- Exhale quickly using abdomen to expel the air
- An audible sound is heard
- This is one round
- 10–20 rhythmical pumps (double the speed of kapalabhati)
- When complete, inhale comfortably
- Engage jalandhara and moola bandha (see page 168)
- Hold for up to 30 seconds
- Release the locks
- Breathe naturally for a few breaths
- Repeat up to 3 rounds
- On completion lie in Savasana (Corpse pose)

Modifications and variations:
- Virasana (hero) or other seated meditation postures
- Use a mat under sitting bones
- Can use a block under knees
- Less pumps
- Less retention
- No retention
- Kapalabhati
- Full yogi breath

Figure 5.10 Alternate nostril breathing – Anuloma Viloma

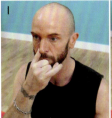 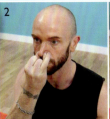 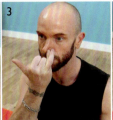 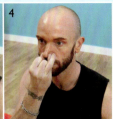 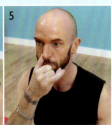

| 1. Close right nostril with right thumb | 2. Both nostrils closed | 3. Close left nostril with ring and little finger of right hand | 4. Close both nostrils | 5. Close right nostril with right thumb |

Purpose: Anuloma Viloma brings balance to the right and left sides of the brain. Daily practice can calm the nervous system.

Benefits:
- Calms the mind
- Provides focus and concentration
- Cleanses the energy channels (Nadis). Ida is cleansed during inhalation (left nostril) and pingala is cleansed during exhalation (right nostril)

Suitable for: Advanced. Supervision recommended.

Precautions:
- Start with smaller breathing ratios, e.g. 1:4, 2:0
- No retention for individuals with high blood pressure, glaucoma, ear or sinus blockage or for pregnant women (inhale and exhale without retention)

Instructions and teaching points:
- Seated in Sukhasana or other meditation posture, body relaxed
- Left hand in chin mudra (see page 164), resting on the knee
- Right hand in Vishnu mudra (see page 164) with right thumb by right nostril
- Right elbow relaxed and into side of body
- Close right nostril with thumb and inhale through left nostril (4 counts) – see photo 1
- Hold breath with both nostrils closed (16 counts) – see photo 2
- Close left nostril with ring and little finger of right hand and exhale through the right nostril (8 counts) – see photo 3
- Keep left nostril closed, inhale through right nostril (4 counts) – see photo 3
- Close both nostrils and hold breath (16 counts) – see photo 4
- Close right nostril with thumb of right hand and exhale through left nostril (8 counts) – see photo 5

Modifications and variations:
- Virasana (hero) or other seated meditation postures
- Use a mat under sitting bones
- Can use a block under knees
- No retention for beginners to this method

MUDRAS, BANDHAS AND KRIYAS

MUDRAS

Mudras are seals or locks. They generally have a purpose of focusing the mind. In Hatha Yoga mudras are said to awaken Kundalini and destroy old age and death.

   Hatha Yoga Pradipika, Chapter 3 vs 5 and 6

The Sanskrit word mudra means: 'gesture', 'attitude', 'lock or seal'. Mudras are yogic positions, usually of the hands and fingers (crossing, extending, touching and bending); but also include eye positions, asanas, bandhas, and breathing and visualisation techniques.

Mudras depict a state of consciousness, but can also develop, and 'lock in', a specific state of consciousness (Hirschi, 2000:2). One simple example of a modern mudra used in the West, would be crossing our fingers, as a symbol to bring luck or a thumbs up to indicate 'well done' (see figure 6.1).

At a basic level, mudras can be a stimulation of pressure points on the hands or body to create energy flow, and/or help bring about relaxation (as used in acupressure, reflexology and meridian therapies). Many mudras have physical benefits as they focus energy on the acupressure points of the hands, thus stimulating certain areas of the body, and can be used to heal physical complaints. They can also alter mood, attitude and perception while deepening concentration and awareness. Mudras are often used during pranayama practices to control the nostril breathing (e.g. chin mudra and Vishnu mudra used with Anuloma Viloma and Nadi Sodhana in chapter 5). These hand mudras work on a subtle level and therefore are considered suitable to be practised and taught early in a student's yoga practice.

Some mudras are considered higher practices, which can awaken psychic powers and Kundalini energy. In Kundalini yoga, mudras are used with asanas to intensify the effects. It is recommended by some schools that these mudras are only taught by an experienced teacher at a time when the

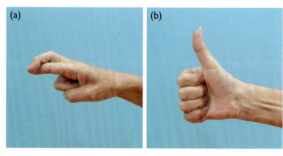

Figure 6.1a and **b** Everyday mudras.

student has reached the appropriate level of self-development, as experience and purity are required for such higher practices, e.g. viparita kirani with mudras and bandhas.

Some of the simple and basic mudras can be practised anywhere – while watching TV or out walking, or while meditating or performing asanas. They can be held for short and longer durations, from a couple of minutes to over an hour in some more specific healing practices.

Different digits (fingers and thumbs) represent different energies (see table 6.1). A knowledge of these energies and the connectedness with other healing philosophies and practices allows experienced persons to develop their own mudras.

Specific texts are devoted to the subjects of mudras, Chinese medicine and healing and other alternative therapies. Readers are therefore guided to further study to develop knowledge in these areas, which are beyond the scope of this book and the current knowledge of the authors.

In summary, mudras, together with the bandhas (discussed later in this chapter), redirect the energy flow, linking the pranic energy with universal force.

MUDRAS AND THEIR MEANINGS

In Hatha yoga, there are many different mudras. Some of the more well-known and commonly practised mudras include the following:

Table 6.1 The connection of mudras to other energy and healing systems and therapies

Finger or Thumb	Ayurveda	Chakras NB: This may differ in some schools of yoga	Palmistry	Connective energy description
Thumb	Fire	Solar plexus	Vital self assertion The will Vitality	Restores balance and equilibrium. The fire energy of the thumb nourishes the energy of the other fingers and absorbs excess energy
Forefinger	Air	Heart	Sense of self-worth Intellectual capacity Individuality	The energy enables us to connect with our innermost being (intuition) and the cosmos/divine energy (inspiration)
Middle finger	Heaven/ether	Throat	Responsibility Initiative Sobriety	Sometimes described as the heavenly finger (Hindu). Mastering the challenges of life
Ring finger	Earth	Root	Relationship to others Ability to love Security	Stamina and staying power Vision for the future Maintains balance in stressful situations
Little finger	Water	Sacral	Communication Creativity Sense of beauty	The realm of the emotions and sexuality Improves mood and raises the vibration of happiness

Adapted from: Hirshchi, 2000

Atmanjali mudra

This mudra, the gesture of prayer, creates harmony, peace, balance and silence by uniting the right and left, yin and yang, masculine and feminine (see figure 6.2). In India this is a gesture of respect and greeting.

- Both hands are placed together at the heart chakra
- Leave a slight gap between the palms
- The thumbs press gently into the breastbone

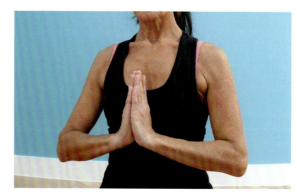

Figure 6.2 Atmanjali mudra

Chin mudra and jnana mudra

The gestures of knowledge and consciousness and the most commonly used mudras.

- Thumb and index finger make a circle and meet at the tips, the thumb symbolises the joining of the divine (thumb) with the individual consciousness (index finger). Depicts the goal of yoga – the unification of Atman (self).
- The other three fingers are relaxed but extended and represent the gunas: tamas (lethargy), rajas (activity) and sattwa (harmony and balance).

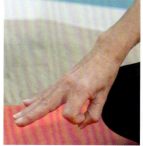 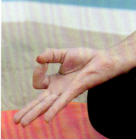

Figure 6.3 Jnana mudra   **Figure 6.4** Chin mudra

When the fingers point upwards, this is jnana mudra (see figure 6.3).

When the fingers point downwards, this is chin mudra (see figure 6.4).

Chin mudra is usually practised at the beginning of the class to symbolise the intention of the aspirant to this union.

The index finger is also known as the ego finger and in chin mudra the ego meets the divine.

Dhyani mudra

The gesture of meditation and contemplation; this is the classic hand position and represents the meditator as being unmoved by their surroundings and immersed in infinite space.

- The two hands make a bowl shape, gesturing that we are open and empty to receive everything we need spiritually.
- The left hand lies in the right with the thumbs touching and pointing upwards (see figure 6.5).

Namaste

This gesture is an acknowledgement of the divine in self and others. In Sanskrit, 'Nama' means 'bow'; 'as' means 'I'; and 'te' means 'you'. Translated, this means 'I bow to you' or 'I see the light in you'.

In certain yogic practices, the thumb is used to massage or stimulate the third eye area, symbolising the divine meeting our awakening point.

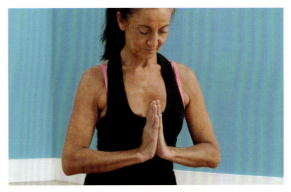

Figure 6.6 Namaste

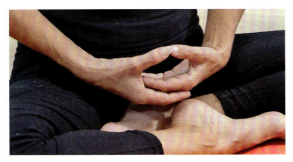

Figure 6.5 Dhyani mudra

The hands are placed together at the heart chakra (see figure 6.2), the head is bowed and the eyes closed. Alternatively, the hands can start at the third eye chakra (forehead, between the eyes) and move down to the heart chakra (chest).

Namaste signifies deep respect. In the West, it is often practised while at the same time, the word 'Namaste' is spoken (see figure 6.6).

One tricks time and obtains qualities like animan, by following his teachings and concentrating on the practice of mudra.
Hatha Yoga Pradipika,
Svatmarama, Ch 3 vs 130

BANDHAS

The word bandha evolves from Sanskrit, and roughly translates to mean: 'lock', 'hold captive' or 'tighten/contract'; which are good descriptions of the physical action of the main bandhas.

Bandhas work in a similar way to mudras, in that they are used to lock in and redirect energy (shakti) for the purpose of spiritual awakening and the awakening of kundalini energy (see chapter 2). Bandhas, like most mudras, are best taught under the guidance of a guru and only at a time of suitable experience, because Kundalini is an incredibly powerful energy. It is recommended that only when an aspirant is ready (after years of yoga practice) should this level of energy work begin.

There are differences and some confusion surrounding the differentiation of mudras and bandhas. In early yogic texts and practices (tantric), both were mainly referred to as mudras, but when Hatha yoga evolved, the techniques were separated and the main bandhas were defined as:

- Jalandhara bandha: throat or chin lock
- Uddiyana bandha: abdominal lock
- Moola bandha: root lock

- Maha bandha or the great lock: when all three bandhas are combined and activated at the same time.

Bandhas should only be practised when the students have achieved a regular yoga practice with purity of mind and body. Examples of how they may be integrated with asana practice are:

- Jalandhara bandha is used during Dwi Pada Pitham/Setu Bandhasana
- Uddiyana bandha can be taught for a brief hold during downward facing dog
- Moola bandha can be taught in meditation pose/cat pose/downward facing dog.

Figure 6.7 Throat/Chin Lock or Jalandhara bandha

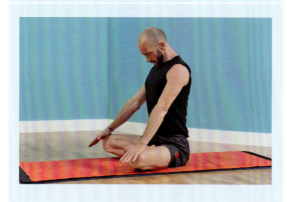

This bandha is considered one to destroy old age and stops the downward flow of prana energy. It also helps prevent headaches and ailments of the eyes, ears and throat through regulation of prana to the head. It is used during Kumbaka (breath retention).

Benefits:
- Brings mental relaxation
- Stimulates throat and thyroid gland
- Helps to regulate metabolism
- Relieves stress
- Relieves anxiety and anger
- Helps develop meditative state

Prohibitions:
- Cervical spine/neck conditions
- High blood pressure
- Heart disease

Instructions:
- Practise on an empty stomach
- Sit in Padmasana
- Hands on knees
- Exhale through the nose
- Lower the head to the chest
- Connect the chin to the notch above the clavicles (the supraclavicular notch)
- Draw the neck up towards the ceiling
- Focus on Ajna chakra
- Retain the breath outside the body
- On slow inhalation lift the chin and sit up tall
- Take a few breaths and repeat

Contracting the throat by bringing the chin to the chest is the bandha called jalandhara. It destroys old age and death

Hatha Yoga Pradipika, Muktibodhananda,1993:352

Figure 6.8 Abdominal lock or Uddiyana bandha

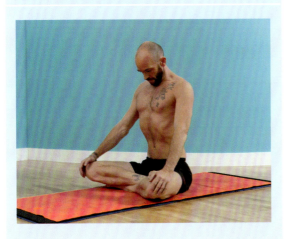

Uddiyana means to fly or to rise up. In this bandha, the abdominal muscles are pulled in and up and this locks in shakti, so it accumulates in this area. This energy/prana (from ida and pingala nadis) is then directed into the Sushumna nadi so it flows upwards to the crown chakra. This takes many years of practice.

> *With the use of this bandha, the great bird shakti (prana) is made to fly up.*
> *Hatha Yoga Pradipika*, 1993:332

Benefits:
- Improves indigestion
- Stimulates digestive fire
- Massages abdominal organs
- Improves circulation to trunk area
- Good for abdomen and stomach
- Relieves constipation

Prohibitions:
- Recent abdominal surgery
- Severe abdominal problems

Instructions:
- Practise on an empty stomach
- Sit in Padmasana
- Hands on knees
- Empty the lungs with a strong forced exhalation through the mouth
- Diaphragm rises out of the way when lungs are empty
- Retain the breath outside the body
- Lean slightly forward
- Activate jalandhara bandha (see figure 6.9)
- Straighten the arms
- Push the knees gently onto the floor
- Contract the abdominals inwards and upwards
- Hold for as long as is comfortable
- Release the abdomen and slowly inhale
- Sitting upright
- Lifting the head

> *Uddiyana is definitely the best of all the bandhas. Liberation will be natural once uddiyana bandha is mastered.*
> *Hatha Yoga Pradipika*,
> Muktibodhananda, 1993:339

Figure 6.9 The Root Lock or perineum/cervix lock – Moola bandha

Through the practice of moola bandha and the pulling upwards of the pelvic floor muscles, apana is prevented from flowing downward.

Instructions:
- Sit in comfortable cross-legged position, preferably Siddhasana
- Gentle yogic breath
- Heel pressed into the perineum/vagina (if possible)
- Contract the muscles of the anal sphincter
- Gently release
- Repeat this practice with a gentle squeeze focusing on the heel of the foot and movement in that area

Intermediate:
- Hold the contraction

Advanced:
- Work with breath retention and other bandhas (under guidance of an experienced teacher)

Press the perineum/vagina with the heel and contracting the rectum, so that the apana vayu moves upwards is moola bandha.

Hatha Yoga Pradipika,
Muktibodhananda, 1993:341

Figure 6.10 The great lock – Maha bandha

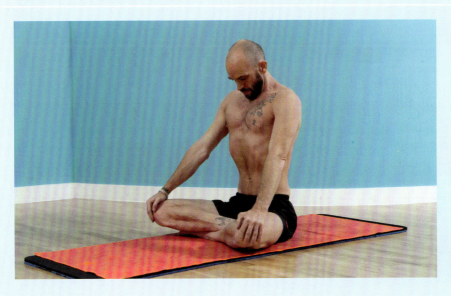

The Sanskrit word, 'Maha' means great. Therefore, maha bandha is called the great lock, because it combines the other three bandhas. When mastered, the great lock is believed to fully awaken prana in the main Chakras (see chapter 2).

Instructions:
- Sit in comfortable cross-legged position (Padmasana, Sukhasana or Siddhasana)
- Press the palms of the hands lightly on the knees
- Relax the body and close the eyes
- Breathe naturally, then exhale forcefully, and completely, through the mouth
- Retain the breath outside. Perform sequentially jalandhara, uddiyana, and moola bandha
- Hold the bandhas and the breath as long as is comfortable, without straining, then release sequentially – moola, uddiyana, and jalandhara bandha
- Inhale slowly
- This is one round
- Relax and let the breath return to normal before commencing the next round
- Work towards three to five rounds

Maha bandha is the bestower of great siddhis.
Hatha Yoga Pradipika,
Muktibodhananda, 1993:302

Maha bandha frees one from the bonds of death, makes the three nadis unite in ajna chakra and enables the mind to reach the sacred seat of Shiva, Kedara.
Hatha Yoga Pradipika,
Muktibodhananda, 1993:302

Maha bandha should not be practised until the other three bandhas have been perfected.

KRIYAS

Kriyas, or Shatkarmas (*Shat* meaning six and *Karma* meaning action) are yogic cleansing exercises which are performed to cleanse the body and assist with the natural removal of waste products (not to be confused with kriya yoga).

Kriyas regulate and balance the production of the doshas (phlegm, wind and bile). It is recommended that kriyas are only practised if there is an imbalance of the doshas (and before pranayama), to remove excess phlegm, wind and bile; as any imbalance potentially leads to disease, (Swami Muktibodhananda, *HYP*,1993:185). If the doshas are balanced, the kriyas or shatkarmas do not need to be practised.

Kriyas are not practised in all yoga traditions, some traditions just use pranayama. A knowledge of the kriyas is useful, just in case they are needed. However, some of the practices (Basti or yogic enema, and Vastra Dhauti or cloth cleansing) are quite extreme and should only be practised under the guidance of a guru while on a sadhana intensive; they are not for everyday practice or for use by the inexperienced!

The six main cleansing practices described in the *Hatha Yoga Pradipika* include:
- Dhauti: internal cleansing (four main areas of cleansing, with a number of different techniques)
- Basti: yogic enema (two techniques)
- Neti: nasal cleansing (four techniques)
- Trataka: concentrated internal (antar) or external (bahir) gazing (two techniques)
- Nauli: abdominal massaging (three techniques)
- Kapalabhati: frontal brain cleansing (three techniques).

Individuals interested in reading more about the kriyas or shatkarmas are guided to the *Hatha Yoga Pradipika*.

JALA NETI (NASAL CLEANSING)

Jala neti is one of the four nasal cleansing techniques. Warm, salt water is used to clean the nasal passages by means of a neti pot (lota). A neti pot is a small clay or plastic container that holds water and has a funnel that inserts in one nostril to facilitate the practice of washing through the sinus passage (see figure 6.11).

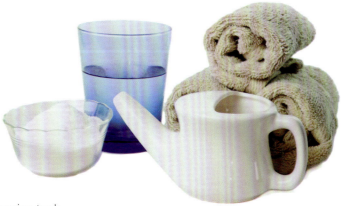

Figure 6.11 Nasal cleansing tools

JIHVA DHAUTI (TONGUE SCRAPING)

Jihva dhauti is one of the many dhautis. Traditionally, the forefinger and thumb were joined to rub the tongue, using a downward action, and then squeeze it, to remove any deposits.

In modern dental hygiene, a tongue scraper (available from most chemists and dentists) can be used to remove bacteria from the tongue; usually in the morning and before bed.

TRATAKA/TRATAKAM (CONCENTRATED GAZING)

Trataka (meaning 'to look' or 'to gaze') practice involves gazing at a point (traditionally the flame of a lighted candle) for as long as is comfortable without blinking the eyes, until tears are shed, to cleanse the eyes.

KAPALABHATI

Kapal means 'cranium' and bhati means 'light' or 'splendour' or 'perception' or 'knowledge', which translates as shining skull. It is an advanced pranayama technique used to cleanse all mucous disorders (see Figure 5.5, page 156)

NAULI (ABDOMINAL CHURNING/ MASSAGE)

The term Nauli, derives from two Sanskrit words: nala and lola. Nala means navel string or tubular vessel, (e.g. the rectus abdominis muscle) and lola means to roll or agitate, (*HYP*.1993:185).

Nauli practice involves contracting and rotating the rectus abdominus muscles to create a churning and massaging effect. It stimulates digestion and positively affects all other disorders of the dosha: massaging and toning the abdominal muscles and internal organs. It generates heat and alleviates constipation.

SESSION STRUCTURE AND GENERAL HATHA FLOW SEQUENCE

7

All Hatha yoga sessions, including large group, small group or one to one personal training sessions and own personal practice, need to have the following structure:
- A preparatory or opening phase
- A main workout phase
- An ending or closing phase

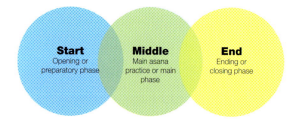

Figure 7.1 Session structure

THE PREPARATORY PHASE

The preparatory phase is the start of the practice or session. It has similar aims to the warm up in other physical movement and exercise sessions, in that it aims to prepare the body and mind for the session to follow. The content of the preparatory phase may vary, depending on the type of session to follow. For example, a dynamic session would have a more dynamic preparatory phase, whereas a restorative session would have a slower and more relaxed start.

Generally speaking, the preparatory phase consists of the following activities, which are by their nature progressive stages for building the intensity. These include:
- An **initial relaxation** component. This will contain relaxation techniques, deep abdominal breathing and full yogic breathing.
- A **mobility or mobilisation** component. This may be performed from any of the following start positions: supine lying, seated, kneeling, standing or any combination of these positions. The start position selected will usually be determined by the position used for the initial relaxation, e.g. if floor lying, then the mobility can also start floor lying, to maintain the flow of the transitions. A mobility component that starts from a lying position, may progress to other starting positions, e.g. lying, seated, kneeling, then standing.
- A **warming** component, such as a sun salutation sequence. Sometimes a collection of other asanas which flow together and develop warmth.

The total time spent on the preparatory phase may take between 10–20 minutes. The specific duration will be dependent on the experience of participants, the activities selected, the temperature of the studio/environment and the content (choice and type of asanas) used in the main phase.

INITIAL RELAXATION

The purpose of the initial relaxation is to relax the body systems and take the focus of the mind away from the trials and tribulations of daily life and bring attention to the 'here and now'. It provides an opportunity to unwind, let go of tension and stress, allow stillness and rest, quieten the mind, focus the breath and allow for fuller and deeper breathing. The aim is not for deep relaxation, thus, the duration is usually around five minutes.

The usual asana for relaxation is Savasana or Corpse pose (see page 134); however, other reclining postures can also be used (e.g. Supta Baddhakonasana or reclined cobbler's pose – see pages 124).

In a colder environment a blanket will be needed to ensure the body does not get too cold. Alternatively, a gentle seated or standing mobility could be used to provide a moving relaxation or meditation. These variations may also be more appropriate for individuals who are not recommended to lie supine, for example: pregnant women (after the first trimester) and also individuals with osteoporosis or individuals who struggle to move from a standing to a lying position (and vice versa).

During the initial relaxation (whether static or moving), each body part can be given attention by using the mind to focus on the area, in turn, each body part can be encouraged to relax and release. Active or passive relaxation techniques or short relaxation scripts can be used (see appendices) to assist static relaxation. For moving or dynamic relaxation, the mind can focus on the moving body part and concentrate on feeling the 'weight' of the movement (light or heavy) and the speed of movement (progressively slower and taking time to slow down).

Deep abdominal breathing (see Figure 5.1), where the tummy rises and falls during inhalation and exhalation can be practised during the initial relaxation. Abdominal breathing is the simplest method of breathing. It brings attention and consciousness to the breath and encourages a deeper and fuller breathing action. Many people are probably not aware of the breath for most of the time and may be more used to the shallow, upper chest breathing, which is common in daily life. Awareness of the breath helps to prepare for the connection of breathing with movement needed during the main phase of the session.

Full yogic breathing (see chapter 5) can also be practised during the initial relaxation. This offers a natural introduction to ujjayi breathing and can be continued throughout the main phase.

MOBILITY OR MOBILISATION – PAWANMUKTASANA

The purpose of the mobility section is to prepare the joints for greater ranges of movement that will happen during the main phase and reduce the risk of injury. Joint mobility exercises warm the joints and stimulate the release of synovial fluid into the joint capsule, allowing them to move more freely and reduce stiffness. In addition, the muscles around the joints are gently lengthened and the mind-to-muscle connection is activated. The duration of the mobility section is usually around five minutes, but in a colder environment, may need to be a little longer.

Maintaining focus on the breath during the mobility section continues to prepare for the movement and breath connection needed for the main phase.

There are a number of start positions that can be used for mobility, these include: lying, seated, kneeling, all fours and standing. The positions selected for mobility will depend on:
- The temperature: in a colder environment, it is better to use positions where more movement is possible to keep warm (e.g. standing or on all fours)
- The preceding activity: if a moving and standing relaxation and meditation is used, then to maintain flow of the transitions, the mobility should start in a similar position
- The ability and needs of the individuals and groups: a group may need to use seated variations to accommodation specific physical or medical needs.

Mobility sequences in different starting positions are discussed later.

BODY WARMING

The purpose of the body warming section is to raise the heart rate slightly, increasing the flow of blood and oxygen to the muscles and raising body temperature and increase breathing awareness, enabling more oxygen to enter and move around the body. The warming section usually takes around five minutes, but may need to be longer in a colder environment.

The warming section also offers a preparation for the mind and an opportunity to rehearse some (not all!) of the asanas that may be used in the main phase. The main asanas that are appropriate will be those that assist with warming, e.g. using the larger muscles of the lower body with a chair, forward bend etc. However, the ability of the group will also need to be considered to ensure a steady and gradual preparation.

The warming section in some styles of yoga (e.g. Iyengar) will be a continuation of mobility to bring warmth and mobility to the joints. The main phase of the session will then continue to build by introducing specific asanas, using props and modifications and steadily building to stronger positions as the session progresses.

Similarly, in a restorative or a relaxed session, any warming activities will maintain the relaxed theme and a floor-based sequence may be continued to maintain the flow within the session.

WARM-UP POSTURES

Figure 7.2 Supine mobilisation

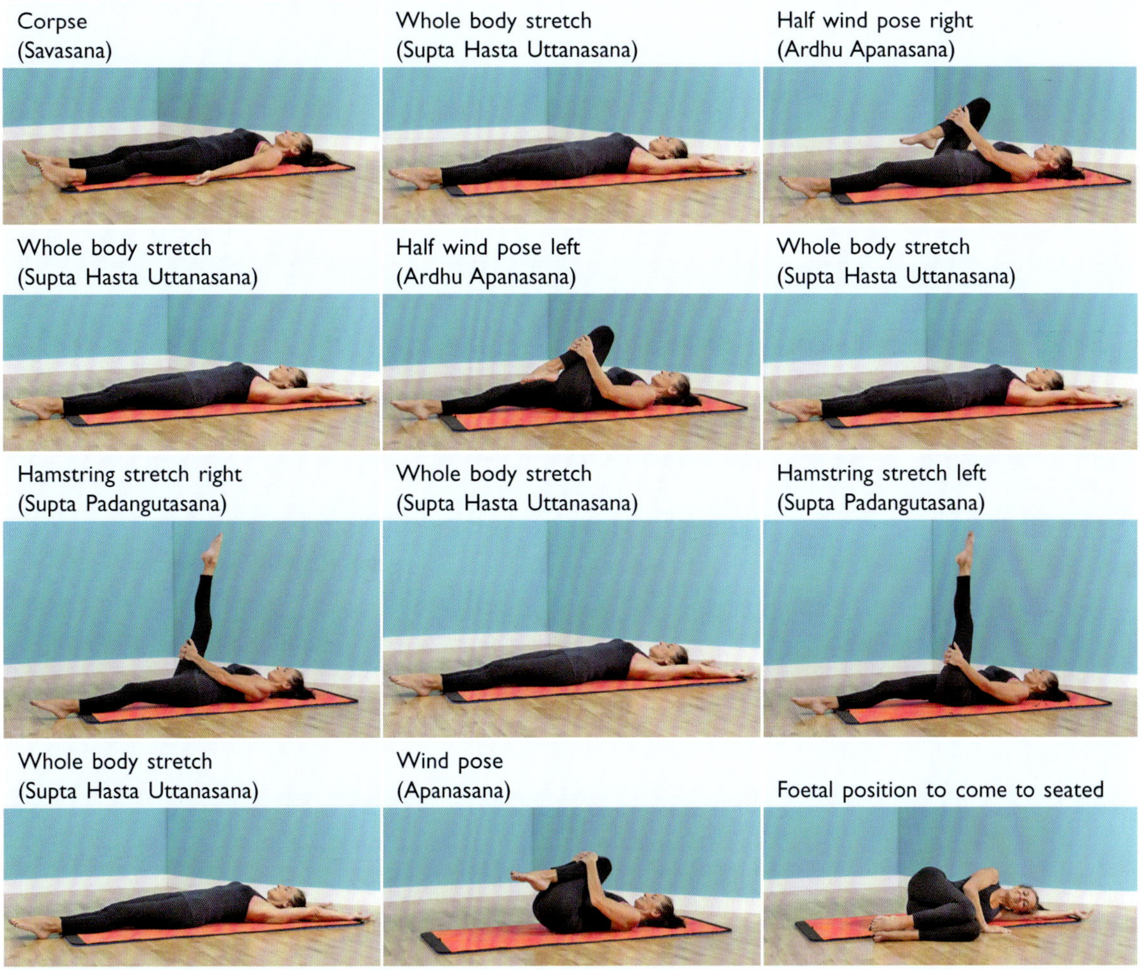

Corpse (Savasana)	Whole body stretch (Supta Hasta Uttanasana)	Half wind pose right (Ardhu Apanasana)
Whole body stretch (Supta Hasta Uttanasana)	Half wind pose left (Ardhu Apanasana)	Whole body stretch (Supta Hasta Uttanasana)
Hamstring stretch right (Supta Padangutasana)	Whole body stretch (Supta Hasta Uttanasana)	Hamstring stretch left (Supta Padangutasana)
Whole body stretch (Supta Hasta Uttanasana)	Wind pose (Apanasana)	Foetal position to come to seated

Purpose: Gentle mobility from initial relaxation

Benefits:
- Mobilise hips, knees and ankle and lower back
- Lengthens hamstrings, gastrocnemius and erector spinae
- Prepares the joints for greater ranges of movement in main session asanas

Suitable for: All levels

Precautions:
- In cold environment, use alternative mobility sequence to generate warmth

Instructions and teaching points:

From Corpse

- Inhale to whole body stretch
  - Both arms float up to floor over head
  - Avoid ribcage flaring and back hyper-extension
  - Extend fingers and toes away from each other
  - Shoulders away from ears
- Exhale to Ardhu apanasana or half wind pose
  - Return arms to side, floating movement
  - Bring right knee towards chest
  - Take hold of shin with hands
  - Soften lower back to floor
  - Shoulders away from ears

Repeat all above on left side

- Inhale to whole body stretch
- Exhale to Supta Padangutasana – hamstring stretch right
  - Float arms over
  - Bring right knee towards chest, holding back thigh
  - Extend knee as far as comfortable
- Inhale
  - Circle ankle one way x 3 times
- Exhale
  - Circle ankle other way x 3 times

Repeat all above with left leg

Repeat whole body stretch

- Exhale to Apanasana – wind relieving pose
  - Bring both knees into chest
  - Breathe comfortably
  - Gently rock side to side
  - Gently rock forward and back
  - Massage lower spine to floor

Figure 7.3 Seated mobilisation

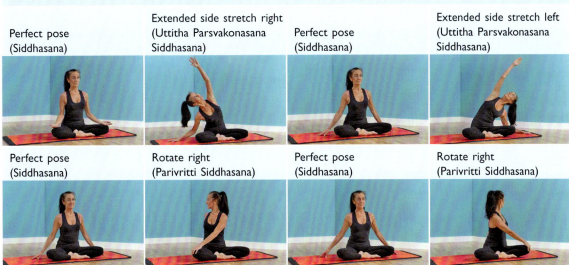

Purpose: Seated mobilising sequence that can be used in preparatory and opening phase

Benefits:
- Mobilises the spine and neck through lateral flexion and extension and rotation
- Improves sitting posture
- Prepares the body for more advanced rotation and laterally extending postures

Suitable for: All levels

Precautions:
- Tight hips or lower back: sit on blocks or use variations
- In cold environment, option to use standing variation

Instructions and teaching points:
In Sukhasana, cross-legged position, sit tall

Seated side bend
- Place the hands about 6-8 inches away from side of body
- Inhale
  - Raise left arm
- Exhale
  - Bend right elbow and extend left arm upwards
- Inhale to lower and release
- Repeat other side

Seated rotation
- Right hand on floor behind back, palm down
- Left hand on floor in front of body
- Inhale
  - Lift body upright
- Exhale
  - Gently rotate to the right
- Inhale to return to centre
- Repeat other side

The sequences can be repeated 2–3 times, increasing range of motion each time

Progressions, modifications and variations:
- Chair seated variation
- Standing variation
- Use other seated posture (perfect pose, lotus etc.)

Figure 7.4 Seated forward bend and Siddhasana Purvottasana

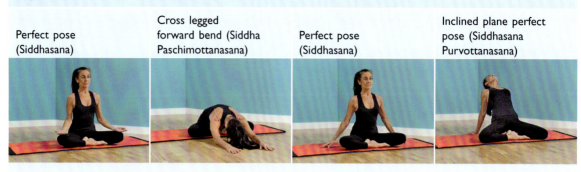

Perfect pose (Siddhasana) | Cross legged forward bend (Siddha Paschimottanasana) | Perfect pose (Siddhasana) | Inclined plane perfect pose (Siddhasana Purvottanasana)

Purpose: Seated mobilising sequence that can be used in preparatory and opening phase

Benefits:
- Mobilises spine and hips
- Opens the hips
- Stretches erector spinae and gluteals (forward bend)
- Stretches hip flexors and abdominals (backward bend)
- Prepares the body for more advanced bending postures

Suitable for: All levels

Precautions:
- Tight hips or lower back: sit on blocks or use variations

Instructions and teaching points:
From Sukhasana

Forward stretch
- Inhale
  - Lift and lengthen spine upwards
- Exhale
  - Lengthen forward, bending from hips and spine into stretch
- Inhale to return to upright seated position

Siddhasana purvottasana
- Exhale
  - Place hands behind back
  - Extend the hips upwards and forwards and lean slightly back
- Inhale to return to upright seated position

Repeat above but with other leg crossed over in front

The sequences can be repeated 2–3 times, increasing range of motion each time

Progressions, modifications and variations:
- Use another seated posture, e.g. Easy or Hero
- Forward bend – hands on floor; elbows on floor; arms extended and forehead down
- Siddhasana purvottasana – small backward lean; raise on to knees and increase lean back
- Repeat sequence with other leg crossed in front and increase range of motion
- Transition to all fours for continued mobility

Figure 7.5 Cat pose or Marjaryasana to Cow pose or Bitilasana
(Mar-jar-ee-AAH-sa-na and Bit-il-AAH-sa-na)

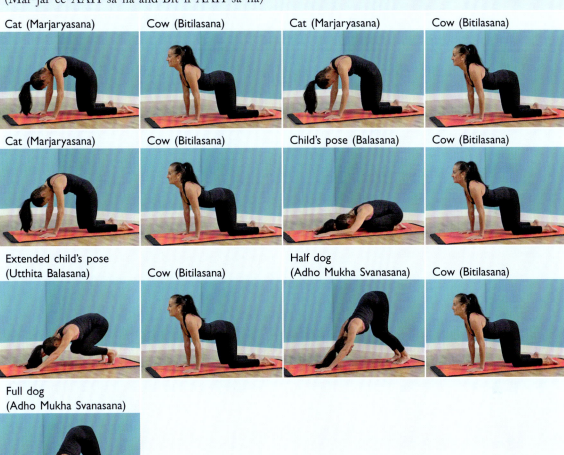

Purpose: Mobilising posture sequence that can be used for preparatory and closing phases

Benefits:
- Mobilises the spine
- Relieves tension in the body
- Prepares the body for larger range of motion flexion and extension postures
- Stretches anterior deltoid, pectorals and abdominals (hollow, cow position)
- Strengthens core (rounded position)
- Stretches erector spinae and gluteals (rounded position)

Suitable for: All levels

Precautions:
- Knee discomfort – knee on blanket
- Back problems – work to comfortable range of motion
- Carpal tunnel syndrome – wrist aligned in fist position or perform standing with hands on thighs

Instructions and teaching points:
Cat
- From all fours
- Exhale
  - Round spine
  - Keep shoulders away from ears
  - Elbows unlocked, toes down
  - Feel tummy button draw towards spine

Cow
- Inhale
  - Hollow spine, looking forward
  - Shoulders away from ears
  - Elbows unlocked, toes tucked

- Repeat sequence 3–4 times to mobilise spine

Progressions, modifications and variations:
- Standing variation with hands on thighs
- Chair seated variation with hands on thighs

Repeat sequence for increased mobility

SUN SALUTATIONS OR SURYA NAMSAKARA

In some hatha sessions, sun salutations – a dynamic sequence of postures performed to flow together from are performed (see opposite). The combination of forward- and back-bending postures generates warmth, as well as mobilising the joints, lengthening the muscles and stimulating and massaging the vital organs of the body. In the initial stages of practice 3–6 rounds may be completed and this can progress to up to around 12 rounds for the more advanced.

However, many of the asanas within the sun salutation sequence require a significant amount of flexibility and some individuals will not have the flexibility to perform the asanas, let alone perform them as part of a dynamic sequence (e.g. sciatica, lower back pain and/or other chronic conditions, restricting mobility). An alternative would be to adapt some or all of the asanas and create a different warming and flow sequence. It could be that just parts of the full sequence are practised (e.g. the first 3-4 asanas) and that these asanas are also modified to achieve a smaller range of motion.

Figure 7.6 Sun salutations (Surya Namaskara)
(SOOHR-ya Nah-mus-KAAHr, Sanskrit origin: Surya – sun; namaskara – salutations)

	Instructions and teaching points:	**Progression/Modification:**
Mountain pose (Tadasana) 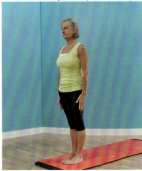		
Arm raise to prayer and slight backward lean (Hasta Uttanasana) 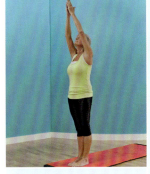	• Inhale to raise arms • Shoulders away from ears • Look up towards thumbs	**Progression**: Increase back-bending range of motion **Modification**: No back bend or backward lean
Forward bend arms extended at side of body (Uttanasana) 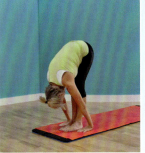	• Exhale • Hinge forward from hips • Abdominals engaged • Lowering chest and chin • Knees slightly unlocked • Open chest wide and arms in crucifix position • Chest towards thighs • Head tucked in towards knees at bottom of movement • Hands on floor at side of feet (can bend knees) • Relax face	**Progression**: Arms extended Legs straight **Modification**: Support body weight with hands on thighs Knees bent Move to a comfortable range of motion Or perform chair pose and then move into forward bend with hands supported on thigh

	Instructions and teaching points:	Progression/Modification:
Eight point salute (Ashwa Sanchalanasana) 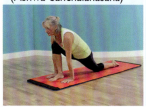	• Inhale • Lunge one leg back • Knee in line with ankle and over toe • Knee down, toe down and look forward • Push through right hip • Back toe points away • Tuck toe under • Retain breath	**Progression**: Larger stride **Modification**: Reduce range of motion
Other leg back – plank (Kumbhakasana) 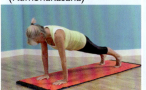	• Breath retained into plank • Elbows unlocked • Bottom in line • Shoulders away from ears • Abdominals engaged • Eyes look to floor • Neck in line	**Modification**: Box position
Chest, chin and knees down (Ashtanga Namaskar) 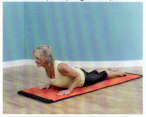	• Exhale • Lower knees, chin, chest down • Concertina spine	**Modification**: Box press to lower and supported slide forward
Cobra (Bhujangasana) 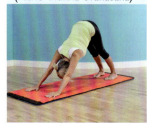	• Inhale • Raise and look forward • Point toes to back of room • Feet open • Gently arch back • Shoulders away from ears • Keep looking forward • Remain engaged in the throat	**Modification**: Sphinx
Inverted V – down facing dog (Adho Mukha Svanasana)	• Exhale • Lift buttocks, abdominals engaged • Shoulders away from ears • Draw tummy button in • Chest through arms, relax heels down • Knees unlocked • Neck long • Eyes look towards toes	**Modification**: Extended child's pose

	Instructions and teaching points:	Progression/Modification:
Leg lunge forward (Ashwa Sanchalanasana) 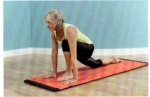	• Inhale • Lunge the same foot forward in-between hands • Look up • Back toe points away • Chest open	**Progression**: Larger range of motion **Modification**: Smaller range of motion Use hand to assist movement of leg into lunge position
Other leg forward into forward bend (Uttanasana) 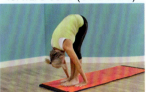	• Exhale • Other leg forward • Hands and feet aligned • Chest on thighs forward bend • Head tucked in • Palms flat on floor where possible	
Raise up, arms overhead into prayer (Hasta Uttanasana) 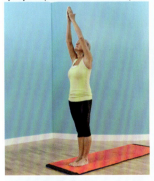	• Inhale • Connect through to crown of head • Hinge upwards from hips • Hands in crucifix • Spine strong • Extended spine to lift • Hands in prayer at top and look up • Extend backwards slightly • Space between each vertebrae	
Mountain pose (Tadasana) 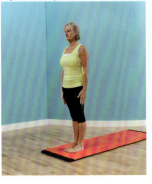	• Exhale • Lower arms and back to sides • Relax into Tadasana	

Purpose: In a physical yoga session, this dynamic series of forward and back-bending postures will mobilise and warm the whole body.

Historically, sun worship has been a part of ancient traditions from all corners of the globe. The ancient Egyptians used their knowledge of the sun and its cycles to build the pyramids, which were aligned for maximum solar radiation. The complex temples dedicated to the sun gods of the Mayans, Aztecs, and Inca peoples divulge comprehensive knowledge of the sun and its cycles. Stonehenge in Britain is considered to have been a stellar observatory to calculate the seasons, equinoxes and solstices. The ancient Chinese philosophers, and Native American Indians both had beliefs based around the sun and its cycles. Sun worship in India dates back to the Vedic period where daily rituals were performed, and still are today, (Satyananda, 1973).

A verse from the Rig Veda states:

We meditate in the adorable glory of the radiant sun. May he inspire our intelligence.

Satyananda, 1973:5

The sequence of postures that are practised today have evolved from solar worship that was not a traditional part of Hatha yoga texts, but was added at a later date. They are a sequence of 12 postures that are considered a sadhana (spiritual practice) unto themselves and consist of vitalising asanas that when practised with pranayama, mantra and meditation can have a powerful effect upon the body and mind, (Satyananda, 1969:153). They have many effects upon the body – muscular, skeletal, internal organs, endocrine system and nervous system, as well as having effects upon the energy bodies, chakras and nadis.

Benefits:
- Increases circulation and blood flow
- Generates heat and warmth
- Strengthens muscles
- Increases energy
- Improves flexibility
- Provides a focus of attention for the mind
- Assists concentration
- Improves co-ordination and balance – motor skills

Suitable for: Intermediate. Can be modified for beginners

Any prohibitions: See prohibitions listed for all postures within the sequence

Precautions:
- Teach stages of the sequence prior to teaching the complete sequence
- Adapt range of motion for different flexibility levels
- Adapt speed of sequence and length of hold in some postures
- Modify postures for different needs and abilities

STANDING EASY SEQUENCE (WARMING)

This sequence is a great warm up in a really cold studio or if you are practising outdoors on a spring morning. It has all the warming elements but omits the inversions and upper body strength work to ensure the body is prepared for this during the sun salutes. Due to its lack of inversions this makes this sequence (if modified in ROM) a suitable warm-up for beginners, and specialised gentler style classes.

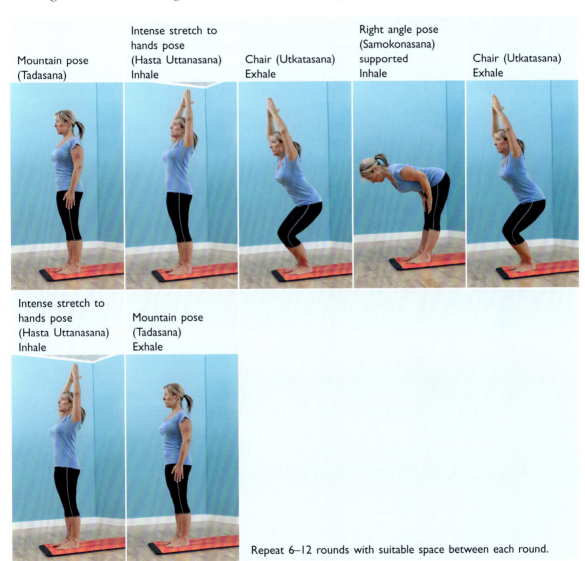

Mountain pose (Tadasana)

Intense stretch to hands pose (Hasta Uttanasana) Inhale

Chair (Utkatasana) Exhale

Right angle pose (Samokonasana) supported Inhale

Chair (Utkatasana) Exhale

Intense stretch to hands pose (Hasta Uttanasana) Inhale

Mountain pose (Tadasana) Exhale

Repeat 6–12 rounds with suitable space between each round.

THE MAIN PHASE

The main phase of practice can be designed in a variety of ways. These include: general hatha, themed sessions, restorative or vinyasa flow.

GENERAL HATHA

In a general hatha session, the asanas are taught individually and postures are selected to provide a whole body and balanced approach. The appropriateness of postures will be selected to meet the needs of the individuals, selected from each of the main groupings and will often include one (sometimes more) postures from the following groups:

- Standing and balancing
- Strengthening and balancing
- Side bending (lateral extensions)
- Forward bends (flexions)
- Backward bends (extensions)
- Twisting (rotations)
- Inversions (the 'upside down' postures, where the head is lower than the heart)
- Seated
- Reclining or lying

THEMED SESSIONS

Some yoga classes have a specialist theme and will consist of a few or a series of asanas from specific groups that will develop a specific theme. Some example themes may include:

- Energising for an early morning session or practice

Theme	Asana		
Twisting	1 Kneeling crescent moon (Anjaneyasana)	2 Crescent moon (Anjaneyasana)	3 Kneeling revolved (Parsva Konasana)
Asana			
Purpose	Prepares lower back	Prepares and warms lower back	First twist
	4 Half lord of the fishes (Arha Matsyendrasana)	5 Bow pose (Dhanurasana)	6 Belly twist (Jakhara Parivritti)
Asana			
Purpose	Second twist	Back bend	Third twist relaxing

- Restorative for a late evening session or practice, e.g. meditation
- Rotation or twisting sequences, performed after a holiday to promote cleansing, e.g. digestion
- A vinyasa flow session with a theme or focused intent, e.g. pranayama
- A flow to match the season – summer, autumn, winter, spring
- A physical focus, such as mobility, strength, core strength, back-bending, chest opening, posture, hip opening, balancing, etc.

RESTORATIVE SESSIONS

In sessions with a restorative theme, the primary focus will be relaxation, meditation, breathing and gentle mobility postures. These classes are often floor based and use postures from the seated and lying groups.

The warm up lying mobilisation sequence is an example of a postures that can be combined and developed in a restorative flow session. An example of this session is Figure 7.2.

VINYASA FLOW

Vinyasa offers a unique way of combining postures, so that each asana flows from one to the other. The flow compares to the movement of the life force; where opposites meet in a flow

Flow sequence	Asana			
Beginner	1 Cat (Marjaryasana)	2 Eight point salute (Ashtanga Namskar)	3 Baby cobra (Ardha Bhujangasana)	4 Extended child's pose (Utthita Balasana)

Postures can be steadily progressed to a larger range of motion, and additional postures can be added or variations of length of hold of each posture can be introduced to develop the flow of the sequence.

| Intermediate | 1 Plank (Kumbhakasana) | 2 Four limbed staff pose – crocodile (Chataranga Dandasana) | 3 Cobra or upward-facing dog (Bhujangasana/Urdhva Mukha Svanasana) | 4 Downward-facing dog (Adho Mukha Svanasana) |

May be practised after sun salutations when the body is warm. The postures can start with a smaller range of motion and no hold, and progress to a larger range of motion and a longer hold. Breath can also be varied. The intensity of flow can be reduced towards the closing phase

of strength, flexibility, movement and stillness.

Vinyasa flow sessions move like a dance, they are rhythmic and create warmth and heat. The sequences are repeated, so that the patterns are imprinted, enabling them to be performed in a trance-like state, giving a feeling of being lost in the moment and at one with the flow. Postures within the sequence are progressively developed to improve flexibility and openness and build a fluidity of movement.

The layering of each posture and sequence has the potential to promote a deep, transcendental approach to practice, where the mind and body are fully immersed in the practice of movement, breath, space and stillness.

The number of postures selected for a flow sequence will depend on the experience of the practitioner and individuals performing the flow.

The timing of the main session is usually around 30 minutes for an hour session, but may be longer if the class is planned for longer. For example a 90-minute session may have a main component that lasts for between 45–60 minutes.

The intensity and complexity of the main session will increase steadily from the opening and preparatory phase, reaching a peak, from which it will steadily decrease, lowering in complexity and intensity towards the closing and ending phase. This graduation of intensity ensures a progressive and layered delivery approach, which enables mixed ability individuals to participate and which minimises the risk of injury and physical stress.

PHASES OF ASANA PRACTICE

Each asana planned within the main session will need to be sandwiched between a preparation pose and a counterpose.

The preparation pose is often an easier or modified version of the full pose and offers a way of preparing the body for the fuller pose. This may be performed as a single pose before the main asana or as part of a sequence of poses (e.g. within a flow session).

The counterpose (pratikriyasana): As explained earlier (see page 59), counterposes re-balance any negative effects of the main asana, they re-balance the physical, mental and spiritual.

Some general guidelines for selecting counterposes are that they:
- Are in the opposite direction of the main pose
- Are easier and gentler than the main pose
- Are specific to the area that may be placed under strain
- May counter the previous movement and link or prepare for the next posture
- Should be mastered before the main asana is practised
- May be performed after a single pose or a sequence of poses
- May be dynamic or static, usually opposite to the main pose (e.g. dynamic to follow static and vice versa)
- Counter the action of the main asana (e.g. for strengthening posture, the counterpose may focus on stretching and vice versa).

For some postures, more than one counterpose may be needed.

For some asanas, another asana is the counterpose, e.g. the head stand potentially creates tension in the neck and the lower back (built up from holding the position); the counterposes could be a shoulder stand to release the tension in the neck and child's pose (balasana) to relieve tension in the lower back.

Other examples of counterposes that are also main asanas include:

Pose	Counterpose
Head stand (Sirsanana)	Shoulder stand (Sarvangasana)
Bridge (Setu Bandhasana)	Fish (Matsyasana)
Single leg forward bend (Janu Sirsasana)	Upward plank, table-top (Purvottanasana)

THE CLOSING PHASE

The closing phase is the end of the session or practice. The purpose of the closing phase is to create the space for a longer and deeper relaxation, meditation practice and more focused pranayama practice (see chapter 5 for breath work and pranayama techniques).

The sub-components of the closing phase are:
- Relaxation
- Meditation
- Pranayama
- Closing prayers or positive affirmations.

The duration of each of the sub-components will be determined by the theme of the main phase. For example, a restorative class will emphasise these components, so they will most likely be longer.

In a more dynamic or themed session, these aspects will still be included, but may be of a slightly shorter duration; depending on the theme of the session.

RELAXATION

The closing relaxation offers an opportunity for deeper relaxation of the mind and body. It allows every cell in the body to assimilate the connection and guidance from the rest of the practice.

A guided relaxation script can be used to assist the connection of mind, body and breath awareness and will also provide a focus that can help to stop individuals from falling asleep.

The usual asana for relaxation is Corpse pose or Savasana; however, other reclined postures, such as Supta Baddhakonasana (page 138) may also be comfortable.

Some examples of relaxation scripts that can be used in their entirety or adapted are provided in the appendix (see appendices).

At the end of the relaxation, an optional short period of silence and stillness can be offered. This can be followed by some lying, mobility activities that progressively bring the body back to a more awakened state and a return to a seated posture, ready for meditation, pranayama and/or prayers/ending affirmations.

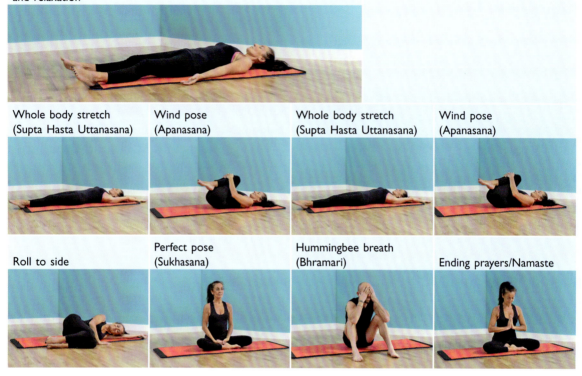

MEDITATION

The heart of yoga practice is to prepare the body, so that the spine is flexible and strong enough (through asana practice) to maintain an upright and seated meditation posture. The usual postures for meditation are Siddhasana or half lotus or full lotus (see chapter 4, seated postures).

Meditation is practised in a seated position to maintain a conscious approach to practice. In the lying postures, there is a risk that individuals will fall asleep, losing the conscious connection to practice. (See chapters 2 and 9 for more on meditation and mindfulness practice). A chair seated position can be used if individuals are uncomfortable in a floor seated position. Alternatively, cushions and blankets can be used to increase comfort in the seated positions (see modifications of seated postures described in chapter 4).

In the ideal floor seated position, the recommendation is for the knees to be lower than the hips, to enable an unrestricted flow of prana (circulation of blood and oxygen).

PRANAYAMA

Pranayama is an advanced technique used within Hatha yoga practice. It should only be practised when fully well (not during illness) and the more advanced pranayama methods (explained in chapter 5) should only be practised under the guidance and supervision of an experienced teacher, and usually on a one-to-one basis, or in small groups.

Beginners or inexperienced individuals are recommended to practise basic breathing techniques, such as abdominal breathing and full yogic breathing (see page 153).

Pranayama and breathing techniques can be practised at both the start and/or at end of a session. One technique that is suitable for practice by most individuals would be hummingbee or Brahmari breath (see page 154). Another technique, for persons with some experience of pranayama practice would be nadi sodhana (see page 155).

CLOSING PRAYERS OR POSITIVE AFFIRMATIONS

There is no single way of closing practice. In traditional practice, the closing offered a way to show respect and devotion to a deity or god/goddess. In 'fitness style' practice, this approach is often modified, to match the comfort levels of Western students and sometimes the closing is neglected, because of this discomfort.

The methods selected to end a group practice will often reflect the values of the individual practitioner and teacher. Chanting, prayers or positive affirmations all offer a way to end the session with appreciation and gratitude, and show respect to the tradition of yoga practice.

Closing prayers or affirmations can be spoken in Hindu or translated. They can be spoken with the hands placed together in prayer position in front of the heart centre/chakra.

Om, Om, Om *Om means 'I am'*
Shanti, Shanti, Shanti *Shanti means 'Peace'*
Om, peace, peace, peace

Namaste

'When you are in that place in you, and I am in that place in me, we are one.'

'With all the knowledge of my mind. With all the force in my hands. With all the love in my heart. I respect the soul within you.'

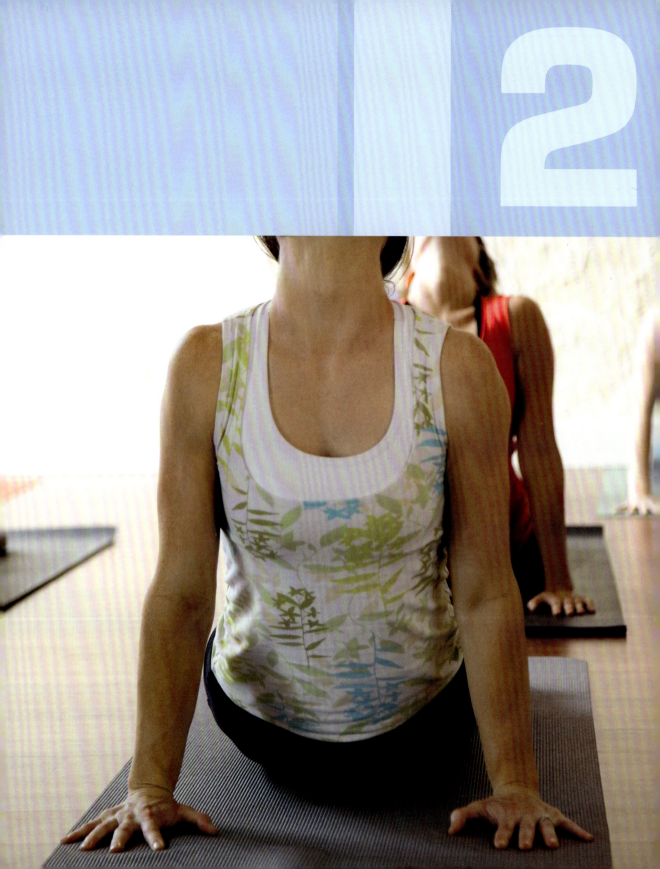

PART TWO

APPLYING YOGA TO MODERN LIVING, AND THE SEQUENCES

The concept of holistic health and well-being or total fitness is recognised in the West and is included as part of the study for many exercise and fitness teacher training programmes. However, the primary focus of the training is on the physiological and physical benefits and how to bring these to fruition.

Yoga in the West is often more about the physical than the spiritual. For most people it is a way of keeping good health and happiness in this busy modern-day world and this is often reflected in the styles of classes available in health clubs and yoga centres alike. Yoga asanas (physical postures) help relieve many symptoms of the stresses accumulated throughout the day, from realigning the posture after sitting at a desk, to releasing the tensions built up through a hectic work and home life, and in relaxing the mind. The relaxation techniques used in yoga take advantage of the limited free time an individual has, and help to concentrate essential 'time to ourselves' in the most efficient and time-saving way. In the age of the twenty-four-hour lifestyle, yoga brings effective methods of relaxation to slow down, relax and unwind, (Satyananda, 1969). This physical, Hatha, aspect of yoga will, for some, bring deep spiritual meaning through learning to listen to the body when in a posture and working with the concentration and control on the breath. However, combining this practice with the disciplines prescribed within the Yoga Sutras of Patanjali (chapter 1) will help prepare the student for higher, more defined practices.

This section of the book explores the concepts of health, fitness, lifestyle and mindfulness and introduces some of the diseases (chronic health conditions) of the modern world and describes how yoga practice and philosophy 'fits' with these concepts and can contribute to the healing process for modern society.

Some Hatha sequences are provided at the end.

YOGA, FITNESS AND HEALTH

MODEL OF HEALTH AND TOTAL FITNESS

The Western model of health and well-being embraces and includes many components of fitness. These are detailed in figure 8.1. Physical fitness (through activity, movement and exercise) is seen as a way of improving and influencing each of the other components.

Physical fitness

Physical fitness is achieved by performing specific types of exercise (walking, swimming, yoga, cycling, gym etc.) in a structured format and at a recommended volume (frequency, intensity, time, type), with the focus towards improving one or more of the five main components of fitness and achieving specific fitness goals. The main components of physical fitness are:

- cardiovascular fitness
- flexibility
- muscular fitness (muscular strength and endurance)
- motor fitness.

Nutritional fitness

Eating a balanced diet containing a variety of foods from all major food groups (carbohydrates, fats, protein, vitamins, minerals, water, fibre),

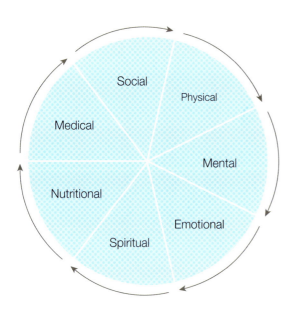

Figure 8.1 Components of health

> By becoming more physically active and connected to the body, we may in turn become more attuned to our nutritional needs and the foods we need to eat to sustain our energy and health.

eaten within current recommended and national guidelines and maintaining a balanced calorific intake to meet energy demands.

Mental fitness
Being aware of the mind and thinking patterns and maintaining positive mental health.

> Physical activity and exercise offer a way of releasing and letting go of physical tension that can be caused by mental stress (fight or flight response), improve self-esteem and reduce the risk of depression. Exercise and activity also offer a way of focusing and distracting the mind from that which it is troubled by (daily problems etc.).

Emotional fitness
Having an awareness of emotions (happy, sad, scared, angry) and being able to manage these and express them assertively with respect for self and others.

> Emotions are a source of energy and exercise and movement offers a way of moving and using this energy, in a positive way. The energy is shifted through movement and does not become stored or blocked, which may contribute to disease.

Medical fitness
Being free from illness and disease and making positive life choices to maintain medical health.

All health white papers of the last decade have included recommendations for increasing physical activity levels and maintaining a level of physical fitness (cardiovascular, muscular, flexibility and motor fitness to help prevent and manage chronic health conditions which are believed to be a major threat throughout the world. The key messages are that to improve health, we need to 'move more often' and 'sit down less'.

Activity guidelines for Adults (19–64) and Older Adults (65+)

- 150 minutes (2.5 hours) of moderate intensity activity accumulated over a week (e.g. 5 days a week, 30 minutes per day, in bouts of 10 minutes or more)

OR

- 75 minutes of vigorous intensity activity
- Include activities to improve muscle strength on 2 days a week
- Minimal sedentary time
- Older adults at risk of falls should include activities to improve co-ordination and balance on at least 2 days a week

(DOH, 2011:7)

Social fitness
Being engaged with community and other people. Being able to create and maintain healthy relationships with others and society.

> Physical activity and exercise offer a way of meeting new people, reducing social isolation and offering structure to the day; all of which improve sense of community and belonging.

Spiritual fitness

Embracing the inner power to create love, peace and live in harmony and balance with self, others and community. Having an awareness of belief systems, which may evolve from family, society, culture and religion, and managing these in a way to make positive decisions for self, others and society.

> Physical activity and exercise improve physical strength and mental and emotional focus, which in turn can improve confidence, self-esteem and well-being and sense of self; which potentially may contribute to changing the way we view the world and how we respond.

PHYSICAL FITNESS

CARDIOVASCULAR FITNESS

Cardiovascular fitness is the ability of the heart, lungs and circulatory system to transport and use oxygen and remove waste products efficiently. It is sometimes referred to as cardio-respiratory fitness, stamina, or aerobic fitness.

Activities to improve this component of fitness are those which use large muscles, in a rhythmic and continuous way and which increase the heart rate at a level that can be sustained for an appropriate duration. These activities may include walking, swimming and cycling, or in a yoga session, a dynamic or flowing sequence of postures, such as sun salutations.

Benefits of cardiovascular training

Regular cardiovascular exercise enables the heart to become stronger, which allows it to pump a greater volume of blood in each contraction (stroke volume). The capillary network in the muscles and around the lungs will increase, which allows the transportation of more oxygen to the body cells and the swifter removal of waste products. The size and number of mitochondria, the cells in which aerobic energy is produced, will increase, enabling increased use of oxygen. Cardiovascular training has a positive effect on overall health and specific benefits include:

- reduce risk of cardiovascular disease (high blood pressure, heart disease and stroke)
- improved cholesterol levels and assist with weight management
- reduce the risk of Type 2 diabetes
- assist stress management and reduce the risk of depression.

FLEXIBILITY

Flexibility is the ability of the joints and muscles to move through their full potential range of movement. It is sometimes referred to as suppleness or mobility.

Activities that improve flexibility are those which allow all the joints and muscles of the body to move through a full range of motion (stretching and mobility). In a yoga session, many of the postures demand high levels of flexibility. The joints and muscles are moved to extended positions. Different approaches to stretching and asana practice include:

- **Static**: where the muscle is slowly lengthened to the end of the range of movement, to a point of mild tension, but not discomfort. This position is then held for a set duration (a number of seconds) and may be repeated 2–4 times.
- **Dynamic**: where the muscle is lengthened to the end of the range of motion, but without the static hold; instead of holding still, the body is moved out of the position and then back into the stretch position for a number of repetitions, progressively stretching further.

In a yoga session, both approaches may be used; this is often determined by the nature of the session – restorative or dynamic.

Benefits of flexibility

Being able to move the joints and muscles through their full potential range of motion is essential for easing the performance of all everyday tasks, such as walking, climbing stairs, bending, reaching or getting dressed. Any loss of mobility or flexibility will have a significant impact on these activities. Being flexible enables movement to be more efficient and contributes to the maintenance of correct posture and joint alignment. It enhances quality of life by maintaining mobility and independence and reduces the risk of injury, especially for older populations.

MUSCULAR STRENGTH AND ENDURANCE (MUSCULAR FITNESS)

A balance of muscular strength and muscular endurance represents a functional level of muscular fitness that is needed to maintain correct posture, perform daily activities (carrying shopping, climbing stairs) and keep the bones and joints healthy and strong.

- Muscular strength is the ability of our muscles to exert a near maximal force to lift a resistance
- Muscular endurance requires a less maximal force to be exerted, but for the muscle contraction to be maintained for a longer duration

Activities to improve muscular fitness are those which demand the muscles to contract to lift a load, which may include body weight exercises or exercise where an external resistance is lifted (gravity or a weight etc.). In yoga most postures, challenge muscular fitness, specifically the standing and balancing, and strengthening postures.

Benefits of muscular fitness training

Muscular fitness training improves the strength and health of the bones and joints and can reduce the risk of osteoporosis and keep the joints strong and stable, reducing the risk of injury. It will improve the tone and shape of the muscles, which can enhance psychological well-being, self-confidence and improve body image. Strong muscles will help to maintain the correct alignment of the skeleton and maintain correct posture. An imbalance of strength in the muscles may lead to postural imbalances, lordosis, kyphosis, flat back etc.

MOTOR FITNESS

Motor fitness is a skill-related component of fitness and refers to a number of inter-relatable factors, which include: balance, coordination, speed, agility, power and reaction time.

Motor fitness requires the effective transmission and management of messages and responses between the central nervous system (the brain and spinal cord) and the peripheral nervous system (sensory and motor). The peripheral system collects information via the sensory system; the CNS receives and processes this information and sends an appropriate response via the motor system, which initiates the appropriate response.

Managing body weight, manoeuvring centre of gravity, coordinating body movements, moving at different speeds in different directions and at different intensities, will all in the long term contribute to improving motor fitness. Motor fitness training can have an indirect effect on other components of physical fitness.

Skilfulness of movement can be lost through the ageing process and through lack of use (inactivity) and may need to be retrained. Learning to balance and coordinate movement patterns takes time and it is essential to break the movement down into its simplest parts and progressively build on these. As a general guideline, starting more slowly with isolated movements and simpler movement patterns, and focusing on correct performance, helps to provide the foundation for developing motor fitness.

PROGRESSIVE APPROACHES TO PRACTICE

Untrained or inactive individuals will need to build up their activity and fitness gradually. Previously inactive people and people with specific joint and muscular problems or chronic health conditions may lack fitness (strength, endurance, flexibility, cardiovascular, skills etc.) and will therefore need to progress steadily and with more guidance from a teacher (observation, correction, teaching to improve their body awareness).

Some general considerations would be:
- Start with a smaller range of motion and build to a larger range of motion
- Use more supportive positions (floor based or more stable base) and progress to more challenging, balance positions, e.g. standing and without support or assistance
- Use props (wall or chair etc) to assist balance or range of motion (cushions and straps etc.) and progress to removing the use of props
- Isolate movements to reduce complexity and work towards combining movements (from static to dynamic practice)
- Use shorter levers to reduce intensity (e.g. bent leg or arm) and progress to increasing lever length (e.g. dancer pose as a quad stretch initially and progress to extending lever away from body)
- Use less repetitions initially and progress to increasing repetitions (e.g. less repetitions of sun salutations or dynamic sequences, progressing to more repetitions)
- Move at a slower pace initially (more static positions) and progress to more dynamic movements.

In a Hatha yoga session, many postures/asanas will need to be modified to accommodate any physical limitations.

LIFESTYLE

Yoga in the twenty-first century is about moderation, or equanimity. The prescribed texts, written by the great yogis, mostly agree that yoga is a practice that can be attained by anyone who chooses to do so, and can be achieved by regularity and moderation. The householder path was prescribed so that the everyday person could have a family, a job, and

Table 8.1 Examples of physical fitness components trained in general fitness sessions and Hatha yoga

Component of fitness	Example of general fitness class activities	Example of Hatha yoga practice activities
Cardiovascular	Dancing, swimming, running, walking, cycling etc.	Dynamic movement sequences, e.g. Ashtanga flow or sun salutations
Flexibility	Static and dynamic stretching and mobility	Asanas that move the joints and muscles through an extended range of motion, e.g. triangle, forward bends, twists, back bends (Cobra)
Muscular strength and endurance	Body weight exercises, weight training, resistance bands, working against gravity etc.	Asanas that require muscle contraction to create a movement or hold a position for an extended duration, e.g. standing balances and strengthening postures, such as warrior, crocodile, plank etc.
Motor fitness	All movements that challenge balance, coordination, speed, power etc.	All postures that challenge balance, coordination, speed, power etc.
Balancing on one leg	Quad stretch	Standing and balancing postures, e.g. tree, eagle or dancer etc.
Coordination to link a series of moves together and move from one position to another	A choreography sequence	Ashtanga flow Sun salutations
Power	Explosive movements and plyometrics	Ashtanga, dynamic yoga

still incorporate yoga practice into his or her life. The four stages of yogic life were set out to allow a full and rich experience that allows us, at the end stages of our lives, to go inward and focus on our spiritual practices, having lived a rewarding life that hopefully made a difference to those people who were intertwined into our tapestry of this incarnation. Surviving modern daily life is a yoga practice unto itself, especially if you live and work in a large city, which can be overcrowded, busy and full of stimulus to distract the senses and confuse the mind. Every day has a new lesson and perspective from which we can grow.

The main aim for the yoga practitioner is to maintain a joyous and moral life without harm to others, or themselves. Some new practitioners of yoga tend to want to rush the process, which was hidden from the everyday person from the great sages for a reason. If the practices are hurried, and the person is not ready, as with everything, things can go wrong. Most yoga practitioners have at some time pushed themselves too far in their asana practice and paid the price with a pulled muscle or a strain. A first-time skier on the slopes who does not want to bother with the beginner's lessons can often pay the price. A person who has not taken driving lessons and thinks they can drive a car would be mistaken. Yoga practices are no different, and to gain the full benefit, the prescribed four stages are the safest, most suitable and satisfying for the average person. It can take many years to cultivate all aspects of yoga, which go way beyond just the asanas. The energy aspects of yoga are considered to be highly evolved processes, which should not be rushed, and should always be guided by an experienced teacher who has gone through the processes themselves and has achieved the aimed results safely.

YOGIC DIET (NUTRITION)

The yogic diet is considered an important aspect of the ways to attain results. The food we eat has a profound effect on our health, both mentally and physically. Certain foods are known to have an effect on our mind and so these foods should be avoided to enhance our practice. Yoga prescribes the following foods to be avoided as they are considered mind stimulants, or go against the Yama of Ahimsa (non-violence).
- Caffeine
- Alcohol
- Garlic
- Chilli
- Meat and fish
- Eggs
- Processed foods
- Old food (i.e. only eat food cooked and eaten that day).

Food is considered, by some, as a pleasure, and while the yogis do not prescribe non-pleasurable activities, they do advocate that food should be fuel for the body rather than something that is craved and over indulged. They also prescribe only two meals a day to allow the digestive system to assimilate and rest correctly. In Ayurveda the digestive fire is known as agni and it is considered a vital part of health. If one has too much fire, assimilation of vital nutrients are passed through the system, which has an effect on our overall health. At the same time if one has a weak digestive fire this can lead to sluggish digestion and constipation which accumulates toxins in the body and leads to ill health in many forms.

Yoga asanas are wonderful for stimulating and balancing the digestive fire and are a very important aspect of the practice. See Shankaprakshalana digestive asana sequence in section 10).

YOGA AND CHRONIC HEALTH CONDITIONS

Yoga offers numerous benefits for improving health on many levels of well-being – physical, mental and spiritual.

PHYSICAL

At a physical level, yoga helps to keep the body strong and flexible and can reduce the physical symptoms of disease. This includes: assisting with pain management, maintaining functional ability and range of motion, improving posture, strengthening muscles and bones.

MENTAL

At a mental level, yoga offers a way for managing the mind. Learning to breathe correctly, to relax and meditate can affect how disease is perceived and experienced; which in turn, can reduce the personal struggle of the ego, against disease (learning to 'let go' of the need to control). The individual can learn to cope with symptoms (e.g. relaxation techniques to assist with pain management and reframing thinking patterns to assist healing).

SPIRITUAL

At a spiritual level, yoga can assist with a reconnection with the aspect of self (higher self, divine etc.) that is accepting, forgiving, compassionate: the aspect that frees the self and others from blame, shame and judgement and accepts the lessons of life (including disease) as part of living.

Asanas/postures help to keep the body flexible, mobile and strong (physical). They help to focus concentration, bringing a sense of alertness and awareness to the mind and a connected and mindful approach to movement (mental). The connection of movement and mind with the breath (the life force) can also help to restore emotional balance. For example, when one is feeling ill or in pain, it is common for the mind to focus on the discomfort and pain, which can magnify these sensations. Mindful yoga practice can help to create an awareness and acceptance of the sensations; limitations in movement are heard and acknowledged, but the concentration of the mind and breath is used to yield with the experience and calm and steady the mind and focus on healing, rather than resisting and fighting against the limitations.

Meditation and mindfulness helps to reduce the clutter of the mind; thought processes can slow down and the mind can become more still and peaceful. When experiencing pain, it is common to freeze-frame the mind and thinking and focus on the painful sensations and its debilitating effects. These thinking patterns will not help the body to heal. Meditation can help to bring the mind to a more calm and peaceful state, where focus on healing thoughts, love and acceptance can be generated. When the mind is relaxed and calm, the body, in turn, will relax. Tense thoughts equal tense, gripping muscles, which block the flow of energy. Calm and steady thoughts will help to relax the muscles, releasing their grip and enabling the flow of energy through the body to be restored.

Breathing/pranayama. The breath is the life force and the practice of full and deeper breathing will deliver oxygen to the body. Full yogic and abdominal breathing also massages the internal organs and helps to relax the body and mind. Alternatively, shallow breathing reduces the flow of oxygen and can create tension and stress in the body. Learning to breath correctly and fully helps to restore the connection between mind, body and the flow of energy. For most health conditions, breath retention should be avoided.

CHRONIC HEALTH CONDITIONS

Some yoga practices, including asanas/postures and pranayama/breathing (Hatha yoga) and even meditation and mindfulness, will need to be modified or adapted for specific health conditions.

A general awareness of the signs, symptoms and physical limitations of some of specific conditions can help to identify postures/asanas that may need to be modified and adapted or in some instances, avoided. Consideration to co-morbid health conditions (more than one condition) and the effects of medication will also need to be given; this information is available in other text books and NHS websites (Patient UK and NICE etc.).

DEPRESSION

A clinical episode of depression is diagnosed when at least two out of three of the core symptoms and three other symptoms are experienced for most of the day, nearly every day, for a minimum of two weeks, (Davies & Craig, 2009).
- **Core symptoms include**: Low mood, reduced interest, pleasure and enjoyment in life, reduced energy and fatigue
- **Other symptoms include**: Feelings of guilt, worthlessness, self reproach; recurrent thoughts of suicide; reduced concentration and attention; low self esteem and self confidence, pessimistic views of the future, decrease in sexual drive, continuing state of worry and apprehension, disturbed sleep (insomnia or hypersomnia); disturbed appetite (poor appetite with weight loss or increased appetite with weight gain); physical inactivity or hyper-activity; thoughts of self harm or suicide (with or without intent).

GENERAL ANXIETY DISORDER (GAD)

GAD is diagnosed when an individual has experienced extreme tension, increased fatigue, trembling, restlessness, muscle tension, worry, and feelings of apprehension about everyday problems, on most days, for the previous six months. The person will be anxious in most situations and there is no known trigger for their experience. GAD is commonly diagnosed with depression, but may also be diagnosed with other conditions, such as alcohol and substance misuse.

Exercise guidance (recommendations and limitations) for depression and GAD

The focus of activity and exercise for clients with mental health conditions would be to:
- Maintain activity levels
- Improve mood, self esteem, confidence and general well-being
- Reduce the risk of other medical conditions that may be caused by inactivity
- Balance energy levels.

General considerations:
- Be considerate, supportive and empathetic to low levels of motivation
- With depression, building motivation to get started is key
- Build up steadily and use an accumulative approach (e.g. a few short practices through the day rather than a long practice) as energy levels may also be low and the person may feel tired a lot of the time. In a session, offer more rests
- Promote enjoyment, fun and pleasure
- Guided relaxation techniques can be useful to provide a focus for the mind and can use language to promote positive self-talk and affirmations (e.g. I give myself permission to relax and be here now; I allow my body to relax and release any tension)
- Use postures that are comfortable for the individual
- Ensure breathing is maintained, avoid holding the breath as this can increase tension
- Avoid breath retention in pranayama
- Use quietening postures for anxiety, e.g. mountain, corpse
- Use re-energising and flowing postures for depression, e.g. slow sun salutations
- Use grounding movements: tree, warrior.

OSTEOPOROSIS

Osteoporosis means 'porous' bones. It occurs when the bones suffer a loss in calcium and other mineral content, which contributes to their becoming thinner, more porous and brittle. This makes the bones more susceptible to breaking (fractures) when put under even minor stress of an everyday bump or fall, which would not affect a person with a healthy bone mass.

Exercise guidance (recommendations and limitations) for osteoporosis

The focus of exercise and activity for individuals with osteoporosis would be to:
- Maintain bone density
- Reduce the progression of the condition
- Strengthen around fracture sites (hip, wrist and spine)
- Maintain mobility and functioning, improve balance and reduce potential risk of falls.

General considerations:
- Avoid forward flexion with or without twisting (some forward bends and triangle etc.)
- Avoid high impact, as these may contribute to vertebral fractures (no jumping to postures)
- Avoid movements which may contribute to trips/falls, e.g. crossing legs when standing (eagle)
- Control neck movements and avoid rolling the neck backwards (some back bends)
- Avoid postures where weight bearing is on the neck area (plough, shoulder stands etc.)
- Include breathing exercises to assist with thoracic spine mobility
- Include pelvic floor exercises
- Avoid lying postures with persons susceptible to vertebral fractures; use standing and seated alternatives
- Ensure environment is free of obstacles to reduce any anxiety about falling
- If weight-bearing exercise is not possible, select chair-based options
- Teach correct lifting technique to assist daily functioning, including how to move safely from standing to floor positions and floor to standing using the support of a chair
- Promote general activity in daily living – walking, gardening, dancing, golf, bowls, standing or sitting with correct posture
- If kyphosis present, avoid head stands or inversions and encourage gentle postures that extend the spine and help to keep upright (Sphinx can help extension and Warrior 2 opens chest).

OSTEOARTHRITIS

Osteoarthritis is a degenerative condition of the joints that is most commonly brought on by the natural wear and tear associated with daily living. The primary joints affected are the weight-bearing joint, which include: knees, hips, lumbar spine, wrists and hands.

The signs and symptoms of osteoarthritis can include: damage to the cartilage, bony growths around the edge of the joint; steady or intermittent pain in the affected joints; discomfort or stiffness when moving the joint; reduction and limitation to range of motion; inflammation and tenderness of the tissues in and around the joint; a crunching or creaking feeling when moving the joint; joint instability and weakness in surrounding muscles; joint deformity.

EXERCISE GUIDANCE (RECOMMENDATIONS AND LIMITATIONS) FOR OSTEOARTHRITIS

The focus of exercise and activity for individuals with osteoarthritis would be to:

- Strengthen around affected joints
- Maintain mobility, functioning and balance
- Maintain activity levels and reduce the risk of inactivity related conditions.

General considerations:
- Avoid excessive repetitions of same joint movement and prolonged activities in the same exercise position, particularly weight-bearing which can aggravate the condition (e.g. holding postures for too long)
- Avoid excessive or fast direction changes (may include sun salutations)
- If joint pain or swelling appears or continues, reduce the intensity (range of motion and weight-bearing) and duration (length of hold) or use a different mode (e.g. in water) or chair based
- Move steadily into and out of postures and avoid holding for too long (avoid jumping into postures)
- Move to a comfortable range of motion
- Use supports and props to adapt postures and range of motion
- Use postures which strengthen affected joints in a comfortable range of motion.

RHEUMATOID ARTHRITIS

Rheumatoid arthritis is an auto-immune and systemic disease that causes chronic inflammation. The joints most affected are the smaller joints of the wrists, hands, fingers and toes, although as a systemic condition, it can affect any organ in the body. In some instances the chronic inflammation can destroy other joint tissues such as cartilage, bone, ligaments and tendons, which causes the joints to become swollen, painful, stiff and sometimes deformed.

RA has periods of remission (when there are no symptoms) and flare up (when the condition is fully active and the body tissues are inflamed. During flare up, signs and symptoms may include: fatigue, loss of appetite, muscle aches, fever, joint stiffness after periods of inactivity (particularly in the morning), red, swollen and painful joints, which in severe cases can become deformed.

Exercise guidance (recommendations and limitations) for rheumatoid arthritis

The focus of exercise and activity for individuals with rheumatoid arthritis would be similar to the guidance for osteoarthritis and includes:
- Strengthening around affected joints (when in remission)
- Maintaining mobility, functioning and balance
- Maintaining activity levels and reduce the risk of inactivity related conditions.

General considerations:
- Avoid exercising the affected joints during a flare-up as this may cause further damage to the joint structure. Gentle mobility may be appropriate
- Be considerate of any past damage to the joints as this may affect the intensity, range of motion and speed of movement that is achievable
- During remission periods work on maintaining strength of muscles around the joint and working through full range of motion.
- Avoid activities that cause pain, excessive repetitions of same joint, high-impact/jumping, stop and start movements, quick direction changes
- Avoid activities using a prolonged one-leg stance. This may include some standing balances (e.g. tree)

- Reduce workload (range of motion, resistance, repetitions) if pain or swelling occurs or use an alternative activity mode, e.g. chair based or water based
- Some exercise positions may not be appropriate, for example resting on all fours will be uncomfortable for wrists (Cat and Cow postures)
- Avoid overstretching and hypermobility – modify most postures
- Exercise in the afternoon or evening to avoid morning stiffness
- Allow an accumulated approach to activity
- Some post-activity discomfort is likely.

NON SPECIFIC LOWER BACK PAIN (OR SIMPLE MECHANICAL LOWER BACK PAIN)

Non-specific lower back pain (LBP) is described as back pain for which the exact cause is not known, but which can usually be attributed to problems with the structures of the spine, (Patient UK, 2012).

Lower back pain can contribute to a significant loss of mobility and restriction of movement that makes daily activities incredibly uncomfortable, painful and much more difficult than usual and may also lead to psychological distress (stress, depression). The pain can vary from severe and long-term, to mild and short-lived. Lower back pain will usually resolve within a few days or weeks for most people; however, episodes can be recurrent.

Exercise guidance (recommendations and limitations) for lower back pain

The focus of exercise and activity for individuals with lower back pain would be to:

- Maintain mobility, functioning and balance
- Maintain activity levels and reduce the risk of inactivity related conditions
- Focus on correct posture and technique
- Lengthen tight muscles and strengthen weaker muscles, that may be contributing to the problem
- Teach spine sparing strategies (lifting correctly, moving from floor to standing, rolling on mats or bed).

General considerations:

- Longer preparatory warm up to allow for gentle mobilisation and progressive increase of range of motion. A longer relaxation period can also assist with a mindful approach to movement and learning about movement limitations and restrictions and how to work within these
- Practise later in the day as the back may be more vulnerable in the morning
- For early practice, the focus should be on very, very gentle mobility and maintaining a correct posture
- Closing phase should emphasise lengthening of tight muscles and promoting relaxation (comfortable positions are needed and may require the use of blankets and pillows to assist relaxation)
- Ensure light engagement of abdominals for all postures
- Use postures which do not overstrain the back – adapt all forward, twisting, lateral and back bends to a comfortable range of motion
- Support spine during forward-bending
- Twist to a reduced range of motion
- Bend to reduced range of motion (smaller range of movement for cobra, cat, upward dog, etc.)

- Avoid extreme bends or twists (e.g. triangle) or modify range of motion significantly
- Avoid high impact (jumping movements), heavy lifting or fast movements as these are jarring
- Avoid trunk exercises during episodes of back pain (focus on abdominal hollowing and light engagement and upright posture)
- Avoid repetitive, fast twisting or bending movements of the spine and exercises that apply a heavy load to the spine, e.g. straight leg forward bends, double leg raising
- Avoid staying in one position for too long
- Gentle mobility and stretching activities for the spine can be performed, modifying the range of movement to suit client needs, e.g. gentle side bends, rotations, pelvic tilts, abdominal hollowing (all fours, prone lying, seated or standing); and Pilates-based abdominal exercises: supine lying heel slides, heel raises, knee raises, reciprocal reach, bridge
- Gentle flexibility exercises for hip flexors, erector spinae, upper trapezius, hamstrings, piriformis, abductors, obliques
- Supine relaxation can be performed with knees bent
- Bridge is great for mobility, but again move to comfortable range of motion.

OBESE AND OVERWEIGHT PEOPLE

Obesity can be defined as a significant excess of body fat that presents an increased risk to health, (WHO, 2012) and other chronic conditions (type 2 diabetes, decreased HDL cholesterols, elevated LDL cholesterol and triglycerides, and high blood pressure).

Exercise guidance (recommendations and limitations) for obesity

The focus of exercise and activity for obesity would be to:
- Maintain mobility, functioning and balance
- Maintain activity levels
- Assist with healthier weight management
- Reduce the risk of other CHD risk factors.

General considerations:
- Consider functional capacity. For example: how easily can they: get out of a chair (sit to stand)? Get up from and down to the floor? How comfortable are they lying or sitting in certain positions? Does body bulk prevent them from performing certain exercises and stretches?
- Aim for lower intensity and impact (no jumping) and where possible non-weight-bearing exercises
- Consider thermoregulation and hydration and possibly exercise at cooler times of day
- Loose fitting clothing should be worn
- The duration of the activity should be built progressively
- Sensitivity should be given to overuse injury risk and precautions taken
- Care with exacerbating any existing joint problems
- Lower intensity (shorter hold and smaller range of motion) as the body-weight is already adding to the resistance being moved
- Slower movements and transitions to allow time for extra weight being moved
- Be sensitive, empathetic and non-shaming.

DIABETES (TYPE 1 AND TYPE 2)

Diabetes occurs when: there is a lack of the hormone insulin and/or the body is unable to respond to the action of insulin; which results in too much glucose in the blood, (NHS Choices, 2012).

Type 2 diabetes develops gradually and signs and symptoms are mild, or absent and can remain undiagnosed for many years. In Type 1 diabetes the symptoms are more obvious and usually develop over a few weeks. These include: excessive thirst, excessive urination, blurred vision, unexpected weight loss (more evident in type 1), recurrent infection such as thrush (more evident in type 2), tiredness.

Exercise guidance (recommendations and limitations) for diabetes

Exercise can benefit insulin sensitivity, hypertension, and blood lipid control. The focus of exercise and activity for diabetes would be to:

- Reduce other cardiovascular disease risk factors linked with diabetes
- Maintain healthy activity levels
- Maintain mobility and functioning.

General considerations:

- Check condition is stable, well controlled and client exhibits no contraindications to exercise (need GP assessment)
- Check client is able to self monitor blood glucose levels and is aware of the effect of activity on blood glucose levels – hypoglycaemia and hyperglycaemia and knows what action to take
- **Do not exercise if**: Blood glucose level is >13 mmol/l and ketone testing is inappropriate or not possible OR blood glucose level is >13 mmol/l with ketones, (Diabetes UK, 2004).
- Encouraging clients to monitor their blood glucose levels before and after exercise and during exercise if the session lasts for more than one hour
- Clients reducing their insulin dose for planned activity/exercise. This will involve some degree of experimenting, as everyone responds differently, it will also depend on the duration and intensity of the activity and the dose and timing of insulin. Advise clients to discuss this with their GP
- Planning exercise 1–2 hours after meals. It is best to avoid exercising during the peak insulin action as this, combined with exercise, increases the risk of hypoglycaemia
- Using injection sites away from areas of the body predominantly used during exercise (usually the abdomen)
- Advising clients to carry fast-acting carbohydrate snacks or drinks when exercising
- Delaying hypoglycaemia can occur up to 36 hours after intense exercise as the muscles refuel. Make adjustments to the timing of exercise or encourage clients to eat a snack before going to bed. This is important if the client exercises in the evening, as there is an increased risk of nocturnal hypoglycaemia
- Being aware that clients with Type 2 diabetes who are not on insulin or sulphonylureas are unlikely to have a hypo; however, they may need to eat soon after exercise
- Making sure that clients drink plenty of water before, during and after activity to avoid dehydration
- Avoiding breath retention in pranayama.

(Adapted from: NICE, 2004 in Lawrence, 2013)

CHRONIC OBSTRUCTIVE PULMONARY DISEASE

COPD is a chronic disabling condition in which the airways and sometimes the lungs themselves have become obstructed (by chronic bronchitis, emphysema, or both), causing persistent and progressive damage which can greatly impair the ability to lead a normal life.

The main symptoms are: a productive cough (coughing up sputum/phlegm); a chronic cough (intermittent or every day); breathlessness that is: worse over time, present every day, worse on exercise, worse during respiratory infections; an increase in chestiness or wheezing during cold weather; peripheral muscle weakness; fatigue.

Exercise guidance (recommendations and limitations) for COPD

The focus of exercise and activity for COPD would be to:
- Manage symptoms of breathlessness and fatigue
- Improve exercise tolerance
- Improve quality of life
- Maintain healthy activity levels
- Maintain mobility and functioning
- Improve efficiency of skeletal muscles to carry out activities of daily living
- Reduce fear, anxiety and depression related to breathlessness.

General considerations:
- Adapting intensity of postures to meet individual needs (range of motion, length of hold, repetitions etc.)
- Encouraging full yogic breath during postures
- Slower and more mindfully focused practice
- Using RPE and breathlessness scale to monitor intensity
- Ensuring optimal medical management and no exercise contraindications
- Ensuring on-going assessment and modification of exercise in response to changes in health status; any significant changes will need to be checked with GP
- Progressing gradually
- Mid-late morning or early afternoon may be best time to exercise due to decreased dyspnoea
- Avoiding exercise in extremes of temperature and humidity
- Avoiding doing too much in one day
- Emphasise optimal posture technique
- If client experiences excessive breathlessness, remain calm and encourage client to adopt a comfortable position and use breathing techniques learned within pulmonary rehabilitation. Leaning forwards, either seated or standing with arms supported, reduces the respiratory effort and will help relax the upper chest while encouraging the use of the lower chest during breathing
- Provide support and encouragement to promote adherence
- Be sensitive to anxiety, fear and depression experienced due to breathlessness and disability
- Avoid breath retention in pranayama
- During closing phase practise relaxation techniques and effective breathing, emphasising the use of diaphragmatic and abdominal breathing.

ASTHMA

Asthma is a chronic inflammatory condition that affects the airways (bronchi) of the lungs. This causes narrowing (constriction) of the airway, which is usually reversible, either spontaneously or with medication, usually an inhaler, (*Patient*

UK, 2011). However, in some people with chronic asthma, inflammation may lead to irreversible airflow obstruction. In asthma the airways are hypersensitive and constrict in response to a trigger, which results in a range of symptoms including shortness of breath, coughing, chest tightness and wheezing, (Lawrence, 2013).

Exercise guidance (recommendations and limitations) for asthma

The focus of exercise and activity for asthma would be to:
- Improve cardiopulmonary fitness
- Maintain healthy activity levels
- Maintain mobility and functioning
- Reduce fear, anxiety and depression related to breathlessness.

General considerations:
- Check the asthma is well controlled and if not, refer the client back to their GP
- Postpone exercise and advise client to visit GP to discuss asthma control: if their sleep is affected by night-time cough or wheeze; their asthma interferes with everyday activities or exercise; their peak flow readings are lower than normal; they are using a reliever more frequently than usual
- Check the client has regular check-ups with GP and has a written personal asthma plan
- A dose of reliever just before exercise may help to prevent symptoms
- Check client has appropriate medications such as inhaler close to hand during exercise
- Teach client to monitor intensity using the RPE and breathlessness scale
- A prolonged warm-up and cool-down will decrease the likelihood of exercise induced asthma (EIA) symptoms developing
- Adapt intensity of postures to meet individual needs (range of motion, length of hold, repetitions etc.)
- Progress gradually
- Best time to practise may be mid to late morning
- Avoid intense practice in extremes of temperature and humidity
- Be aware of environmental triggers such as hot or humid days when ozone levels are high, or cold air. Use a scarf to cover the mouth and nose during cold weather
- An interval approach to exercise, where periods of aerobic activity are interspersed with short breaks, is less likely to provoke EIA
- Make sure you know how to manage an asthma attack
- Avoid breath retention in pranayama
- Be sensitive to anxiety, depression and fear in response to breathlessness and disability.

HYPERTENSION

Hypertension is sometimes referred to as the 'silent killer' as most people with hypertension feel well and are symptom-free (asymptomatic). If someone has really high blood pressure they may get headaches, but this is unusual. Other possible symptoms include sight problems, nosebleeds and shortness of breath, (NHS Choices, 2010).

Exercise guidance (recommendations and limitations) for hypertension

The focus of exercise and activity for hypertension would be to:
- Maintain cardiopulmonary fitness
- Reduce associated and modifiable risk factors
- Maintain healthy activity levels
- Maintain mobility and functioning.

General considerations:
- Ensure client checks with GP and is on appropriate medication before beginning practice. **Do not exercise if**: resting blood pressure is >180/100 mmHg
- Encourage appropriate breathing technique
- Discourage isometric activity (e.g. holding postures for too long), high intensity or sustained upper body exercise due to the possibility of an excessive increase in blood pressure
- Some postures will be contraindicated (inversions)
- Range of motion should be adapted to accommodate individual needs
- Avoid breath retention in pranayama
- Transitions to floor and standing will need to be slower (may need to avoid or adapt sequences, e.g. sun salutations).

YOGA PHILOSOPHY IN MODERN LIVING

The philosophies, ideas and instructions of the ancient yogis offered great wisdom on many aspects of living including how to live a happy life, how to stay healthy, how to find inner peace and live peacefully. This knowledge is still relevant in the modern world, although some of the teachings and practices may need to be 'modified' to fit with more modern lifestyles and the world we live in.

The main aim of yoga is to find a way back to the ultimate reality. The idea is that the world we live in is not the total sum of our existence. The concept of yoking or uniting infers that we are separate, or have been separated from something, and this separation contributes to distress and disease. Yoga philosophy, teachings and the many traditions and approaches within yoga aim towards an awareness and exploration of this 'separateness'. The age-old questions of 'who am I?', 'what is my purpose?' and 'where do I go once I leave this body?' have been asked since the beginning of time. The yoga journey is one that enables a return to the united and connected state.

What must be considered is that many of the ancient teachings were written in Sanskrit and through translation, teaching and reprinting, the original meanings may have been lost or misinterpreted. In many ways, any attempt to offer explanation can only be an estimate and partial representation. However, what can be respected is that the many philosophies and ideas from the many and varying paths, schools and disciplines of the yoga traditions offer the opportunity to find peace and happiness. There is no dogma, just the joy of practice.

An awareness of those things that potentially disturb our peace is the first step to finding a way to resolution. Yoga offers this.

THE SENSES

The senses (taste, touch, sight, hearing and smell) are considered the gateway of pleasures. The modern world offers a constant barrage of material aspirations through advertisements, and bombardment of a whole array of new and exciting ways to find pleasure, which can lead our senses (and subsequently the mind) to attach to things that are transient and fleeting. This in turn can lead to a habitual desire for more, which in turn can lead to dissatisfaction, as once the sensory pleasure has been appeased, the mind then wants more, and what was once a delight, may become the 'norm'. These habits can lead to pain as the need to replenish the excitement of the initial aspiration becomes harder to achieve, and in extreme cases could become an addiction.

Yoga teaches us contentment (Santosha) in life that helps to reduce these wants and needs, which can ultimately cause pain and disappointment (addiction to suffering).

THE MIND

In the modern world, there are so many ways for the mind to become distracted (mobile phones and Internet advances etc.) and overstimulated. These distractions offer interruptions and can prevent us from being totally 'in the moment', fully experiencing the here and now, which is what true yoga represents. The past cannot be changed, and the future cannot be dictated, the only thing that is real is the present. A wise teacher once said 'the greatest *gift* of life is the *present*', which is why it is called the 'present'.

Overstimulation of the mind can lead to a never-ending source of inner chit-chat that can become overwhelming and lead to many varying mental disturbances, including stress, anxiety and depression. A key consideration for the modern world is that depression is predicted to become the second leading contributor to the global burden of disease by 2020 (World Health Organisation).

The yoga philosophies and activities of focusing the mind whether through asana practice (chapter 4), meditation (chapter 2), mindfulness (chapter 9) selfless service (discussed on page 215), or devotion through chanting (mantras, chapter 2) allows the mind to steady and find a central point of focus, which in turn, can lead towards finding an inner quietness and peace; away from the external stimulations of the modern world. Within these various practices of taming the mind, there develops a natural joy of life that is simple and natural. The notion that we are human beings and not human doings is a part of the yoga philosophy.

DEVOTION

For the ancient yogis, devotion and worship of a deity was a key theme. This tradition of taking time out from one's day to worship or pray is still relevant today. It can be incorporated into modern lives by simply setting aside time to meditate or be mindful (if the devotional aspect of yoga is not your leaning).

The final three limbs of Ashtanga Yoga are collectively known as Samyama, the practice of concentrating and immersing ourselves in an object. The object could be a natural environment, a walk in the park or by a river, or it could be focusing on a picture (see chapter 2).

STAGES OF LIFE

The yoga tradition respects different stages of life and ageing (chapter 9). The tradition of the householder path takes us through the natural cycle and allows us the gift of time in this world to have a family, work at a job we care about, and advance ourselves as a whole person.

Yoga practices offer a joy of life that can be passed onto our families, and in the final stage we can leave our loved ones behind and seek spiritual involvement with the knowledge that yoga has made us a better person, who may have made a difference in the world in some small way.

ADAPT, ADJUST, ACCOMMODATE

There is a yoga philosophy of 'Adapt, adjust, accommodate', which offers an alternative perspective to one's outlook on life. It explains that the ego is the base of many of our pains and suffering, the idea that we are right and others/everything else is wrong can lead us to wanting the world and the people around us to change to suit our own ideas, wants and needs.

Within the idea of 'adapt, adjust, accommodate' we release ourselves from our ego and stop trying to control everything and everyone around us. The moment we just adapt ourselves to a situation that we cannot change we let go of the possible negative outcomes.

For example: imagine you are stuck on a train and late for a very important business meeting; the frustration (of the ego) builds the longer the train sits on the track. You keep asking the conductor 'when will we be moving'? The train conductor cannot give you a time, as the cause for the delay is uncertain and out of his control. The rising frustrations lead to anger which has physiological effects: blood pressure rises, the pulse quickens, the breath becomes rapid, anxiety rises, hormones fly through the body as adrenalin begins to soar etc. The cascade of reactions brought on by the mind (and thinking) leak into every cell and have an immediate and lasting effect on you (fight or flight response), over something you have no control of. Regardless of how important the meeting is, the external situation cannot be changed and the reality is that it is rather pointless to allow yourself to let this external and unchangeable situation cause so much internal turmoil; and in the long term contribute towards many potential health risks – both physical (heart attacks, hypertension etc.) and mental (anxiety and depression).

The moment we step back and look at the situation as an observer and realise we are not in control of what happens externally, we can adapt, adjust and accommodate. We may not be able to change the external, but we can manage and change the internal response. If we do this, all the frustration and anger can fade away and we can regain peace.

Adapting, adjusting and accommodating offers a way for reviewing and revising our whole outlook on life. We let go of the thing we cannot control and manage the things we can control (how we respond). External changes and stress become less and less of a problem.

ACCENTUATE THE POSITIVE

Chapter 2 verse 33 of the Yoga Sutras of Patanjali teaches us to cultivate the opposite of the mind's disturbance; it is called *'prati paksha bhavana'*. This practice teaches us to avoid undue pain by trying to see the positive in what the mind has connected as being negative. This can be difficult, however, if coupled with 'adapt, adjust, accommodate' this practice can become easier.

Often in life, if things do not turn out how we want or how we expect, there can be suffering and turmoil, created by the mind and the way we think; we judge the situation as negative or bad. However, in many instances there is a lesson and sometimes not getting what we think we want brings something more pleasant.

The aim is to let go of what we perceive as being negative; you never know what is around the corner.

For example: your car doesn't start in the morning and you will be late for an important meeting. The mind perceives this as bad which creates chaos and turmoil. But look at this in a different light: it could be that this occurrence prevents something else from happening (e.g. an accident). Alternatively, you may miss an opportunity you wanted and perceived as being good for you. The point is that the mind attaches and judges (good or bad), so rather than flowing with different life experiences, we allow it to create pain and suffering. The aim is to 'let go' of the experience and 'let it be', 'let things unfold'.

There is nothing good or bad, but thinking makes it so.

Shakespeare

BHAKTI YOGA IN MODERN LIFE – CHANT AND BE HAPPY

The foundation of Bhakti yoga is humility, and this is considered the easiest path to the Divine (Sivananda, 1964). In modern life, daily chanting assists the mind in becoming focused and can help bring an inner peace and happiness with very little effort, just devotion and faith. Within Hinduism, and therefore many yoga traditions, salutations to a chosen deity are at the heart of every spiritual enactment, from going to temple to the rising of the sun.

One of the earliest mantras found in the Vedas is that of the mantra to the sun called the Gayatri mantra. Many scholars have written many interpretations of the Sanskrit words. The mantra is said to be recited at the early dawn just prior to the sunrise until the full orb is visible on the horizon. It is prescribed in the scriptures that the mantra is recited as often as possible during this time period and is said to bring spiritual knowledge and a long and auspicious life, (Feuerstein, 2003:300).

Whatever the mantra chosen to recite in the day it should be either chosen by yourself because it calls to you from the heart, or given to you by a spiritual guru. It can be recited mentally for

The mantra is:

Om bhur bhuvah svah
Om tat savitur varenyam
Bhargo devastya dhimahi
Dhiyo yo nah pracodayat

George Feuerstein in his book *The Deeper Dimensions of Yoga* translates the mantra to mean:

'Om. Earth. Mid-Heaven. Heaven. Let us contemplate the excellent splendor of God Savitri, so that he may inspire our contemplations'.

a deeper effect and in this way can be used in a public place to help bring quiet and solitude. Many yoga traditions chant when they are preparing and cooking food to instil the power of the mantra into the food that is to be eaten.

Bhakti yoga is devotion and so should be performed with love and not for the sake of thinking it will attain any spiritual realisation. Sound is vibration and those sounds can be uplifting at every level from the mental through to the physical cellular structure. Dr Masaru Emoto wrote of his experiments in his bestseller *The Hidden Messages in Water*, where he viewed and recorded water samples at the microscopic level and then again after chanting words such as Hate and Love to different bottles. The results showed a vibrant white microscopic image for those chanted with love, yet in contrast the water chanted with hate showed a black and spikey microscopic result, (Emoto, 2005).

SERVE, GIVE, LOVE IN DAILY LIFE

The four paths of yoga advocate devotion, service, meditation and study as the ways to attain yoga. The Yoga of Service, or Karma yoga, is often the hardest to fit into a modern householder lifestyle, as time seems to be an ever increasingly difficult thing to find. Swami Sivananda says in his book *Bliss Divine* that life is meant for service and those who give selflessly shine the Divine light, (Sivananda, 1964:383). The selfishness within ourselves becomes selfless through *seva* (Sanskrit for service) or Karma yoga. Egoism, anger, hatred and jealousy, as well as ideas of grandeur, are removed, (Sivananda, 1964). Swami Satyananda equates Karma yoga to a moving meditation, where the aspirant is busy doing, however their focus is eka grata (one pointed) in contemplation of the higher reality.

The action of doing for others brings many things to the mind to disengage the senses and allows focus to control the thoughts that have arisen in contemplation of all that is, at that moment, (Satyananda, 1980). Within the act of Karma yoga we engage our passion for ahimsa (non-violence) by acknowledging that we are doing our very best, without any reward, (Satyananda, 1980). Discrimination between what we need in life and what we want helps bring clarity and inner peace as the ego becomes tame and quiet and with each selfless act comes a little more peace, (Satyananda, 1980).

In modern life there are many opportunities for selfless service through helping our families and friends in times of need. Integrating charitable work, from sponsored events to regular voluntary work, or offering to cut an elderly neighbour's hedge once in a while, is Karma yoga in action.

A starting point for Karma yoga would be to engage yourself in each individual task, whether that is about yourself or not. For example, next time you eat a meal simply spend the 20 minutes or so to eat it with no other distractions. Taste every mouthful, feel every chew, smell every smell and immerse yourself in what you are doing. Appreciate that someone grew this food for you, which they picked for you to buy. Imagine how many people and animals are involved in creating this beautiful food for you to prepare. Enjoy the idea that you created this meal along with condiments from around the globe, such as the oil and salt, and think about how many continents and people were involved in bringing that sea salt and olive oil to your kitchen. As you prepare the food think about how the power gets into your home ready to cook and imagine who had made the knife you use to cut and the board to chop on. Where did all this come from? Yes, you bought it but someone else brought it to you. By thinking about all this and then enjoying every mouthful, we begin to open our eyes to what is beyond ourselves. It can be easy to believe the world is all about us.

Begin with appreciation for our lives, and then move into appreciating and helping others. From the odd charity donation comes a firm commitment and a sponsored run or swim, and then a voluntary afternoon helping out. One day this could all lead to total selfless service.

GRATITUDE – GIVING THANKS

Be thankful for everything! Start the day giving thanks and end the day giving thanks.

By this means you will acquire the glory of the whole world.

The Emerald Tablet, (circa 5000–3000 BCE) in Byrne (2012)

When you open your eyes in the morning, be thankful for another day of life and breath. Be thankful that you had a bed to sleep in and a roof over your head. Be thankful that you can lift yourself out of bed and move to other rooms in the house. Be thankful for every item in the home (toothbrush, toothpaste, towels, kettle), be thankful for the food in your cupboard, that you have crockery and cutlery to eat with. Be thankful for the money to pay bills. Be thankful for the work you do, be thankful to the people who provide services that you use. Be thankful for electricity, gas, fresh water etc. The more thankful we become of everything we have, the more this grows and expands. A recommended text for building gratitude is *The Magic* by Rhonda Byrne.

AN OUNCE OF PRACTICE IS WORTH A TON OF THEORY: JNANA YOGA IN MODERN LIFE

The path of Jnana yoga, or study and knowledge is considered to be fruitful but one that should be taken with caution. The idea that yoga can be attained through reading and study alone is not necessarily true. The practice of integrating the knowledge learnt and using it for sadhana (spiritual practice) is sometimes easier said than done. There are many people capable of reading the scriptures and repeating them verbatim, however, living the yoga is a very different matter. As with any yoga practice or path it is the living in the everyday moment that is the challenge, and all the reading and study in the world does not make a yogi. Swami Sivananda remarks that even the naked sadhu who shows the world his non-attachment by having not even clothes to wear and just his hands for his begging bowl, may be the biggest scoundrel who has internal attachments that no one can see. He also states that the yogi who lives in the bustle of the city with fashionable clothes may have the least attachments or cravings and yet can still live and work in the modernised world, (Sivananda, 1964). Jnana yoga is the path that helps to bring mental nudity, a purity of the internal state. External signs of a yogi are not a certainty to authenticity, (Sivananda, 1964).

Bringing Jnana yoga practice to life in modern-day living is difficult to achieve, as there are few opportunities to spend our days debating, discussing or studying yoga philosophy. Our studies are our own and not a conversation starter to illicit an expected show of interest from friends or new acquaintances. Yoga philosophy is not something that should be offered in daily conversation to those who are innocent of its wonder. The jnana gained from study is not to be offered in bite-size chunks to impress or bemuse. The yogi who uses his knowledge for any other means than sadhana, has missed the point completely, and is not practising with the right dharma (intention). Only the very wise can keep such knowledge to themselves and for themselves. Every action has a reaction even through speech, and karma incurs from every thought or deed that has been ignited by our words. The jnana for you may be the distraction for someone else that has heard your snippet of the scriptures and has no other wisdom to back up the countering thoughts that have been stirred. The path of Jnana yoga is a solitary one and therefore quite a tough one to follow.

An easier path to follow is the collection of Raja, Karma and Bhakti yoga. Integrating selfless service, chanting, meditation, asanas and Ashtanga yoga into modern life allows us to maintain balance and equality in practice. Our bodies stay fit and healthy with no distraction from disease and pain through Hatha practice. Our minds become calmer and able to cope better in the face of diversity through pranayama and meditation practices. Remembering the Yamas and Niyamas helps us be a better person with a kind heart and sympathetic ear. Service to others from simply washing the dirty dishes without want for reward (usually in praise) or helping a sick friend can build within us the joy of giving. Chanting the mantras while performing our duties will enhance the vibration of everything in our lives, from the food we cook and eat, to the job we do. Shining the light of yoga comes through action and not speech. Be the yoga rather than brag about it. Use the jnana and radiate a special attribute to the world that comes from the collective yoga practices.

MINDFULNESS

Mindfulness has its roots in both ancient Buddhist and yoga practices, including meditation and modern psychological techniques, such as cognitive behavioural therapy (CBT). In recent years, there has been an increase in the scientific evidence to support the benefits of mindfulness as part of the healing treatment for many physical illnesses (chronic pain, hypertension etc.) and mental health conditions (stress, anxiety, addictions, eating disorders etc.) (Mental Health foundation, 2010).

The reported benefits of mindfulness practice include:
- Greater insight
- Improved problem solving
- Reduced anxiety and depression (neurosis)
- Less self-judgement, berating and blame
- Enhanced self-esteem and confidence
- Reduced chronic pain and physical distress
- Reduced use of pain-related medication and drugs (including self-medication and addictions)
- Improved sleep quality
- Decreased blood pressure
- Increased vitality and enjoyment of life
- Greater mind and body integration
- Increased blood flow
- Reduced risk of CHD
- Improved resilience and ability to cope
- Improved well-being (mental and physical).

Mindfulness is an integrative mind and body technique that helps to focus attention on the 'here and now', the present moment. It involves building a conscious awareness and acceptance of thoughts and feelings as they surface, without judgement or attachment, so that rather than becoming enmeshed in every stirring and sensation, one is more able to detach and notice what is happening and make new choices.

Mindfulness offers a way for becoming an observer of experiences, rather than having to be a part of every story (drama, adventure, thriller, fairy tale, musical etc), that the mind is able to create from different life experiences.

Mindfulness involves:
- **A**wareness and acceptance: noticing the thoughts and sensations that rise from an experience
- **B**eing with and braking: learning to say 'stop' to the inner monkey and chatterbox
- **C**hoosing to change: consciously making new choices for self.

As figure 9.1 illustrates, mindfulness practice is a way of making the mind a best friend, rather than an enemy.

Activity

- Prepare for a five-minute mindful practice. Find a quiet space, choose a focus object or sound and prepare to either sit comfortably for 5 minutes or walk slowly for 5 minutes (choose the latter, if stillness feels unnatural or uncomfortable)
- Centre your attention by focusing awareness
- Consciously scan your thoughts, body sensations and feelings as they arise with an open mind, shifting freely from one perception to the next
- No thought, image or sensation is considered an intrusion, just notice them
- Stay here and now, with a 'no effort' attitude
- Use the focus object as an 'anchor' to the present, if the mind wanders or becomes enmeshed
- Let go of any need to analyse or fantasise regarding any of the contents of awareness
- Be with the experience
- Notice

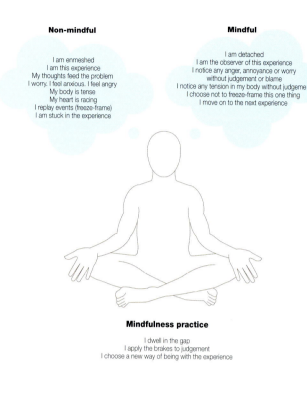

Figure 9.1 Mindfulness

An analogy could be watching a movie. If you freeze-frame the movie at a specific point (or your mind and thoughts on a specific experience), then all you will see is that one screen shot in your mind. Alternatively, you can choose to notice the need to attach to a specific thought and instead of freeze-framing, let it pass and let it go, letting the movie of the mind continue to play and move on to the next experience.

As with other meditation practices, a focus or attention point can be used for when the mind wanders or drifts. The focus point may be:

- An object (a candle, a picture, a mandala, a statue of a deity, a crystal)
- A process (the breath)
- A sound (mantra)
- A physical movement (e.g. each step of a walk)
- A visualisation (focusing internally on something that makes you feel warm inside).

Learning to be mindful is a journey that requires ongoing attention and practice. It may be more effective to have the guidance of a therapist, who can help with developing a sense of non-judgement and acceptance of the journey. The aim of practice is to learn how to take and apply mindfulness to all experiences of daily living.

YOGA SEQUENCES
by Conrad Paul

SHANKAPRAKSHALANA – DIGESTIVE CLEANSE SEQUENCE

Shankaprakshalana is a digestive cleansing sequence usually performed twice a year at an ashram and under the guidance of a guru and prescribed conditions. Translated, shank means 'conch' which is said to represent the coiled shapes of the intestinal tract, and Prakshalana means 'to wash thoroughly'. The purpose of the practice is to wash the whole digestive tract and purify the body both physically and energetically.

Shankaprakshalana is a series of asanas performed on an empty stomach. The asanas performed in the sequence activate peristalsis (digestive tract contractions to increase movement) and progressively open each area of the digestive system and its sphincters to allow for a complete cleanse.

Prior to performing these asanas, salt water is drunk and after the asanas, evacuation (excretion) is performed. After the initial cleanse a special meal known as *Khicheri* is consumed, consisting of boiled rice, lentils and ghee (clarified butter) which helps to prevent intestinal cramps and allows for the purification to continue without any adverse side effects. This is followed by adequate rest and a specific diet for one month to complete the whole sequence of practice.

A simpler version known as Laghoo or short Shankaprakshalana can be performed once a week and does not entail the specific diet regime, (Satyananda, 1976:484).

An adapted version is provided here to enable yoga teachers to help students initiate a healthy digestive system. The designed sequence consists of a series of forward-bending and twisting asanas, back bends and finishes with some simple inversions to encourage digestive health and regulate Agni (digestive fire).

The sequence *does not* involve the drinking of salt water or evacuation after the asanas. The asanas maintain the theme of intestinal massaging and manipulation; but the aim is for the sequence to be accessible for individuals within the modern yoga studio environment.

A recommendation to drink herbal teas and eat simple healthy foods is offered after the sequence. The sequence is a very popular one that is often taught before and after the more indulgent festivals such as Christmas and Easter when people tend to eat much richer food than normal, however it can be taught at any time of the year (see page 220 for sequence for digestive health).

Table 10.1 — Sequence for digestive health

For intermediate to advanced practitioners, who have developed their strength, flexibility and cardiovascular fitness

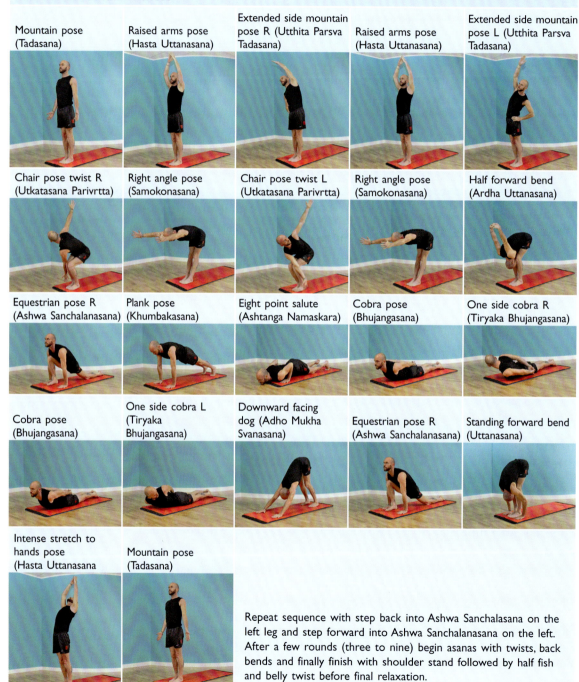

Repeat sequence with step back into Ashwa Sanchalasana on the left leg and step forward into Ashwa Sanchalanasana on the left. After a few rounds (three to nine) begin asanas with twists, back bends and finally finish with shoulder stand followed by half fish and belly twist before final relaxation.

HIP OPENING SEQUENCE – PREPARATION FOR MEDITATION POSES

Table 10.2 — Hip opening sequence – preparation for meditation poses

Expanded mountain (Prasarita Tadasana)	Expanded hands up (Hasta Prasarita)	Expanded to foot (Prasarita Padottonasana)	Expanded plank (Prasarita Khumbakasana)	Expanded salute (Prasarita Namaskara)
King Cobra (Raja Bhujangasana)	Extended mountain pose (Prasarita Parvatasana)	Expanded to foot (Prasarita Padottonasana)	Expanded hands up (Hasta Prasarita)	Expanded mountain (Prasarita Tadasana)

Prasarita means to expand or spread. The whole sequence works in a similar way to Surya Namaskara, but with the legs wide to open the hips and inner thighs. As Raja yoga is one of the four paths of yoga it is understood that the hatha practices help in freeing energy and train the mind to be able to focus through movement into stillness. Those who can sit comfortably in Padmasana, Siddhasana, or Sukkhasana, which require freedom in the hips and back area, can gain the acknowledged benefits of meditation.

Following asanas (counterposes) to balance the sequence would be:
- Garudasana
- Hasta Padangustasana
- Raja Kapotanasana
- Simhasana
- Gomukasana

SALUTE TO LORD SHIVA

This sequence takes reference from Lord Shiva in his destruction phase and his cosmic dancer pose. In his role as destroyer Shiva is called Rudra, hence the posture is called Rudrasana. This sequence can be taught as a standing warming sequence before or instead of Surya Namaskara.

It is suitable for advanced practitioners who have developed their flexibility, strength and cardiovascular fitness.

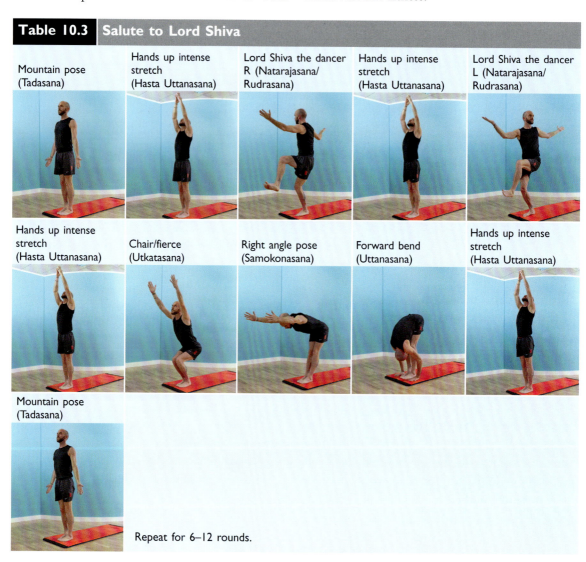

Table 10.3 Salute to Lord Shiva

Repeat for 6–12 rounds.

STRENGTH SEQUENCE

This sequence is a salutation that incorporates the Crow for upper body strength and mental concentration. For those unable to practise the Crow they should stay in Malasana for the breaths allotted to the crow. The one-footed chataranga is performed to the breath count and not rushed. When taking the one footed Down Dog the leg lifts as you push into the pose, not after you get there although this can be done as a variation.

Table 10.4 Strength sequence

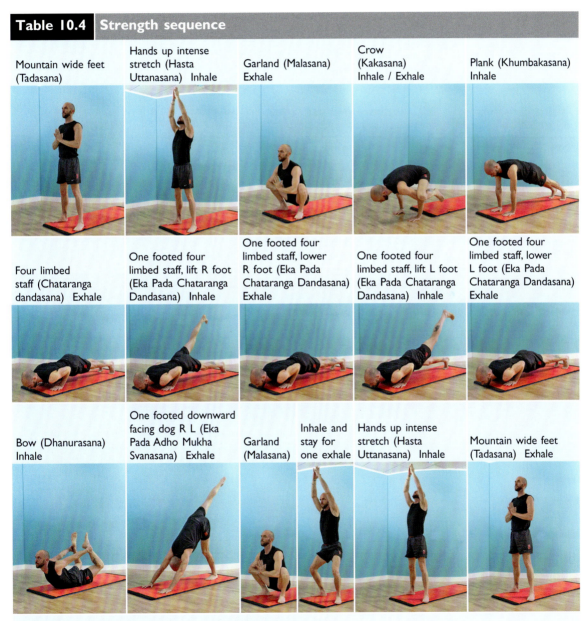

Repeat for 6–12 rounds with suitable space between each round.

FOCUS SEQUENCE

This sequence is a standing balance sequence that brings focus. Each posture moves seamlessly from one to the other without putting the foot down until the second Hasta Uttanasana. At first the sequence is difficult to maintain without balance issues but with perseverance and repetition it becomes a flowing dance of concentration and beauty.

Table 10.5 Focus sequence

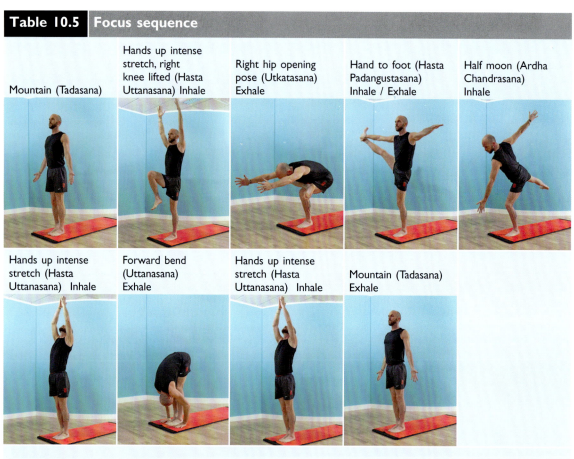

Repeat both sides for 6–12 rounds with suitable space between each round for rest and contemplation. The sequence can be added to and combined with other vinyasa flow sequences.

PREPARATION FOR MEDITATION SEQUENCE

This sequence is a seated mobiliser of the hips, legs and spine and is a late evening practice to prepare the body for evening meditation. A suitable daytime practice before meditation would be Surya Namaskara or asana practice.

Table 10.6 Preparation for meditation

Staff (Dandasana)	Toe bending (Padanguli Namana)	Ankle bending (Goolf Naman)	Ankle rotation (Goolf Chakra)	Knee bending (Janu Naman)
	Inhale / Exhale • as you bend and flex the toes	Inhale / Exhale • as you point and flex the foot from the ankles	Inhale / Exhale • as you rotate 3x each direction each breath – same then opposite	• Exhale, slide knee to chest • Inhale, slide leg back to start
Janu Naman and Chakra sequence	Half butterfly pose (Ardha Titali Asana)		Wide-legged forward bend (Upavishta Konasana)	Meditation pose (Sukhasana with chin mudra)
• Exhale, slide knee to chest and float out to the floor	• Inhale, lift knee back to bodyline and slide away • Exhale, cross one foot up to opposite thigh area as if going into half lotus pose, • as you breathe gently draw the knee to the floor and release to mobilise the hip		• Inhale, open legs as wide as comfortable • hinge from the hips and bring chest towards the floor	Choose a posture that suits you today

Repeat both sides for 6–12 rounds with suitable space between each round for rest and contemplation. The sequence can be added to and combined with other vinyasa flow sequences.

SEATED MOBILISATION WITH AFFECTION SEQUENCE

This sequence is simple yet powerful. It allows us to bring warmth and support into an area we have possibly not focused on for a while.

At birth, the neck is unable to support the head for a few months. Whenever your parents held you in their arms they had one hand under the back of your head for support. Those three months or so of being held and supported had a profound effect on us for our entire lives. Try to remember the last time someone touched the back of your head? It is a very intimate area and one that is only touched with permission. The memories of being a baby may not be vivid, however, the emotion and memory is there.

Table 10.7 Seated mobilisation with affection sequence

Seated cross-legged position	Hands behind the head	Gently reach over to one side Exhale	Back to centre with hands still in place Inhale	Gently reach over to one side Exhale
Back to centre with hands still in place Inhale	Turn and fold towards the right thigh Exhale	Lift up back to centre with hands still in place Inhale	Turn and fold towards the left thigh Exhale	Lift up back to centre with hands still in place Inhale
Place hands behind back on the floor and do a gentle backbend				

Repeat two or three times. If the lateral extension pose needs to be supported, one hand goes to the floor for support with the other hand behind the head – change hands as you change sides.

REFERENCES

Alidina, S., *Mindfulness for Dummies*, John Wiley & Sons Ltd., West Sussex, 2010

American College of Sports Medicine (ACSM), *Guidelines for Exercise Testing and Prescription* 8th ed. Lippincott, Williams & Wilkins, Philadelphia, 2010

Arnold, Sir, E. (trans), *The Bhagavad Gita*, Duncan Baird Publishers, London, 2005

Benson, H., *The Relaxation Response*, Avon Books, New York, 1975

Bloom, W., *The Power of Modern Spirituality: How to Live A Life of Compassion and Personal Fulfilment*, Piatkus, London, 2011

Bradshaw, J., *Homecoming: Reclaiming and Championing Your Inner Child*, Piatkus, London 1990

Buddhananda, S., *Moola Bandha: The Master Key*, Bihar: Yoga Publications Trust, Bihar, 1996

Byrne, R., *The Magic*, Simon and Schuster, London, 2012

Chanchani, S., Chanchani, R., *Yoga For Children: A Complete Illustrated Guide To Yoga*, UBS Publishers' Distributers Pvt. Ltd., New Delhi, 1995

Chopra, D., *The Seven Spiritual Laws of Success*, Bantam Press, London, 1996

Chopra, D., *Perfect Health*, Harmony Books, New York, 1991

Dana Akers, B., *The Hatha Yoga Pradipika: The Original Sanskrit Svatmarama*, YogaVidya.com, New York, 2002

David Coulter, H., *Anatomy of Hatha Yoga*, Body and Breath Inc., USA, 2001

Davies, T. & Craig, T. eds., *ABC of Mental Health*, 2nd ed. BMJ Books, West Sussex, 2009

Department of Health, *Be Active, Be Healthy*, 2009. Accessed on: 5-6-2011 from: http://www.dh.gov.uk/prod_consum_dh/groups/dh_digitalassets/documents/digitalasset/dh_094359.pdf

Department of Health, *Start Active, Stay Active*, 2011. Accessed on: 18-2-2012 from: http://www.bhfactive.org.uk/userfiles/Documents/startactivestayactive.pdf.

Desikachar. T.K.V., *The Heart of Yoga: Developing a Personal Practice*, Inner Traditions International, USA, 1999

Devereux, G., *Dynamic Yoga*, Thorsons, London, 1998

Durstine, L. J. et al, *ACSM's Exercise Management for Persons with Chronic Diseases and Disabilities*, 3rd ed. Human Kinetics, Champaign, 2009

Ellesworth, A., *Anatomy of Yoga*, Hinkler Books, Australia, 2010

Emoto, M., *The Hidden Messages In Water*, Atria Books, New York, 2005

Feltham, C. & Horton, I. eds, *Handbook of Counselling & Psychotherapy*, Sage Publications Ltd., London, 2000

Feuerstein, G., *The Deeper Dimension Of Yoga: Theory and Practice*, Shambhala Publications, London, 2003

Feuerstein, G., *The Yoga Tradition: In History, Theory And Practice*, Hohm Press, Arizona, 1998

Forstater, M. & Manuel, J., *The Spiritual Teachings of Yoga*, Hodder & Stoughton, London, 2002

Gross, R. & McIlveen, R., *Psychology: A New Introduction*, Hodder & Stoughton, London, 1998

Harris, A. and Harris, T., *Staying OK*, Arrow Books, London, 1995

Harrision, E., *Teach Yourself to Meditate*, Judy Piatkus (Publishers) Ltd., London, 1993

Haywood, S. and Cohan, M., *Bag of Jewels*, In Tune Books, Australia, 1992

Hay, L., *You Can Heal Your Life*, Hay House Publications, USA, 2005

Hirschi, G., *Mudras: Yoga in Your Hands*, Weiser Books, USA, 2000

Iyengar, B.K.S., *Yoga: The Path to Holistic Health*, Dorling Kindersley Ltd., London, 2001

Jeffers, S., *Feel the Fear and Do it Anyway*, Arrow Books, London, 1987

Jeffers, S., *Feel the Fear and Beyond*, Rider, London, 1998

Karmananada, S., *Yogic Management of Common Diseases*, Yoga Publications Trust, Bihar, 1983

Keane, S. & Hedrén, T. *Seasonal Pilates*, UK, 2011. Available from: www.seasonalpilates.com

Lawrence, D., *The Complete Guide to Exercise Referral*, Bloomsbury, London, 2012

Lipton, B.H., *The Biology of Belief: Unleashing The Power Of Consciousness, Matter And Miracles*, Hay House, London, 2005

McLeod, J., *An Introduction to Counselling*, 3rd ed. Open University Press, Buckingham, 2003

Mental Health Foundation, *Mindfulness Report*, Mental Health Foundation, London, 2010

Millman, D., *Way of the Peaceful Warrior*, New World Library, California, 1984

Millman, D., *Sacred Journey of the Peaceful Warrior*, New World Library, California, 1991

Millman, D., *No Ordinary Moments*, New World Library, California, 1992

Millman, D., *Wisdom of the Peaceful Warrior*, New World Library, California, 2006

Mindell, A., *Sitting in the Fire: Large Group Transformation Using Conflict & Diversity*, Lao Tse Press, Portland, 1995

Myss, C., *Why People Don't Heal and How They Can*, Bantam Press, London, 1997

NHS choices, *Hypertension*, 2010. Accessed on 12-4-2012 from: http://www.nhs.uk/Conditions/Blood-pressure-(high)/Pages/Introduction.aspx

NHS choices, *Eatwell Plate Guidelines*, 2011. Accessed on 12-4-2013 from: http://www.nhs.uk

National Institute of Health & Clinical Excellence (NICE), *Type 1 Diabetes in Adults: Understanding NICE Guidance*, NICE, London, 2004. Accessed on 15-10-2005 from: www.nice.co.uk

National Institute of Health & Clinical Excellence (NICE), *Chronic Pulmonary Disease In Adults In Primary And Secondary Care*, NICE, London, 2010. Accessed on 24-3-2012 from: http://www.nice.org.uk/nicemedia/live/13029/49425/49425.pdf

National Institute of Health & Clinical Excellence (NICE), *Hypertension – Clinical Management of Hypertension in Adults*, NICE, London, 2011

National Obesity Observatory, *Measures of Central Adiposity as an Indicator for Obesity*, National Obesity Observatory, UK, 2009

Ornish et al, *Intensive Lifestyle Changes May Affect The Progression Of Prostate Cancer*, trial report, 2013. http://www.easybib.com/kb/index/view/id/58

Pascal, E., *Jung to Live By*, Souvenir Press, London, 1992

Patient UK., *Asthma*, 2011. Accessed on: 8-4-2012 from: http://www.patient.co.uk/health/Asthma.htm

Patient UK, *Non-Specific Lower back Pain*, 2012. Accessed on: 23-3-2012 from: http://www.patient.co.uk/health/Back-Pain.htm

Patient UK, *Hypertension*, 2012. Accessed on 28-4-2012 from: http://www.patient.co.uk

Peale, N.V., *The Power of Positive Thinking*, Cedar, London, 1953

Prabhavananda, S. & Isherwood, C., *How to Know God: the Yoga Aphorisms of Patanjali*, Vedanta Press, California, 1953

Raven, H., *Crystal Healing: A Vibrational Journey Through the Chakras*, Raven & Co., UK, 2000

Ramaswami, S., *The Complete Book Of Vinyasa Yoga*, Marlowe and Company, New York, 2005

Ramaswami, S., & Hurwitz, D., *Yoga Beneath The Surface*, Marlowe and Company, New York, 2006

Rieker, H.U., *The Yoga of Light*, The Dawn House Press, USA, 1971

Rinpoche, S., *The Tibetan Book of Living and Dying*, Rider Books., USA, 1992

Rogers, C., *On Becoming a Person. A Therapist's View of Psychotherapy*, Constable & Co. Ltd., 1967

Roger, J. & McWilliams, P., *You Can't Afford the Luxury of a Negative Thought*, Thorsons, London, 1990

Scott Peck, M., *The Road Less Travelled*, Routledge, UK, 1978

Sharamon, S. & Baginski, B., *The Chakra Handbook*, Lotus Light Publications, USA, 1991

Skynner, R. & Cleese, J., *Families and How to Survive Them*, Vermillion, London, 1983

Steiner, C., *Achieving Emotional Literacy*, Bloomsbury, London, 1997

Stevens, A., *Jung: A Very Short Introduction*, Oxford University Press, Oxford, 1994

Stewart, I. & Joines, V., *TA Today: A New Introduction to Transactional Analysis*, Lifespace Publishing, Nottingham, 1987

Swami Muktibodhananda, *Hatha Yoga Pradipika*, Yoga Publications Trust, Bihar, 1993

Swami Muktibhodhananda, *Swara Yoga*, Yoga Publications Trust, Bihar, 1984

Swami Saradananda, *Chakra Meditations*, Watkins Publishing, UK, 2010

Swami Satchidanada, *The Yoga Sutras of Patajali: Translation and Commentary*, Integral Yoga Publishing, USA, 1990

Swami Satyananda, *Asana Pranayama Mudra Bandha*, Bihar, 1969

Swami Satyananda, *Surya Namaskara, A Technique of Solar Vitalisation*, Yoga Publications Trust, Bihar, 1973

Swami Satyananda, *Meditations from the Tantras*, Yoga Publications Trust, Bihar, 1974

Swami Satyananda, *Sure Ways to Self-Realisation*, Yoga Publications Trust, Bihar, 1980

Swami Sivananda, *Bliss Divine: A Book Of Spiritual Essays On The Lofty Purpose Of Human Life And The Means To Its Achievement*, Divine Life Society, Rishikesh, 1964

Swami Sivananda, *Raja Yoga*, Divine Life Society, Rishikesh, 1986

Swami Sivananda, *The Science of Pranayama*, B N Publishing, 2008

Swami Vivekananda, *Raja-Yoga*, Ramakrishna-Vivekananda Center, New York, 1956

Swami Yogakanti, *Sanskrit Glossary of Yogic Terms*, Yoga Publications Trust, Bihar, 2007

Tiwari, M., *Ayurveda Secrets of Healing: The Complete Ayurvedic Guide To Healing Through Panch Karma Seasonal Therapies, Diet, Herbal Remedies And Memory*, Lotus Press, Wisconsin, 1995

Waugh, A. & Grant, A., *Anatomy and Physiology in Health and Illness*. 11th ed., Churchill Livingstone, Edinburgh, 2010

World Health Organisation, *Obesity Factsheet no. 311*, 2011. Accessed on 2-3-2012 from: http://www.nhs.uk/Conditions/Obesity/Pages/Introduction.aspx

World Health Organisation Website, *Depression*, 2012, Accessed on 2-1-2013 from: http://www.who.int/mip2001/files/1956/Depression.pdf

Zinker, J., *Creative Process in Gestalt Therapy*, Vintage Book, New York, 1977

GLOSSARY OF TERMS

Auto-immune diseases Diseases that cause the body's immune system, which normally fights foreign substances such as viruses and bacteria, to attack other tissues in the body because they identify them as foreign tissue (e.g. rheumatoid arthritis)
ABPM Ambulatory blood pressure monitoring
Abhinivesa One of the klesas. Attachment. The source of fear
Ahimsa One of the yamas. Love. Non-violence to yourself or others, in thought or deed
Asana One of the eight limbs of yoga, focusing on positions or 'postures', as practised within Hatha yoga
Ajna Chakra Third eye chakra located between the eyebrows. Energy or command chakra
Anahata chakra Heart chakra – located at the heart centre, spiritual heart chakra
Anga Limb – as in the eight limbs of yoga
Ananada Bliss state
Anandamaya kosha The most important of the five sheaths or layers of the astral body. The sheath of bliss
Annamaya kosha One of the five sheaths or layers of the astral body. The anatomical sheath
Antaraya An obstacle or obstacles to a stable and clear mind and mental state
Anuloma Viloma Alternate nostril breathing – pranayama technique
Apana Prana energy located in the abdomen. Waste or dirt. The centre where waste collects and where elimination is dealt with
Apana-vayu The aspect of prana that is responsible for excretion
Aparigraha Yama (restrictions); non-receiving of gifts (bribes)
Artha Purpose or meaning
Asana Postures, positions or poses
Ashram Spiritual retreat, monastery
Ashtanga Eight limbed. Described by Patajali in the Yoga Sutras
Ashtanga yoga One approach to Hatha yoga, developed by Pattabhi Jois
Asmita One of the kleshas. Sense of ego
Atman Individual spirit or the self (see also Brahman)

Asteya One of the yamas. Not coveting that which belongs to others
Avatar Manifestation of god in physical form
Avidya One of the klesas. A state of delusion, ignorance and lack of wisdom; which Patanjali suggests is due to the ego drive within the mind to pursue selfish desire
Ayama Extension of energy

Bahya Exhalation
Bandha Locks or seals
Bhagavad Gita Part of the Mahabharata, text where Krishna teaches yoga to Arjuna
Bija mantra Seed. Syllable that contains specific power
Brahaman Supreme spirit, Divine, God – the unchanging self, eternal self aspect (see also Atman). Absolute reality, supreme reality. Infinite and eternal, all-pervading, one and indivisible
Brahmacharya One of the Yamas. Celibacy. Movement towards highest modification of the senses

Chakra Wheel or vortex. The astral centres of the body, critical junctions (located along the spine). When activated by asana and pranayama chakras transform cosmic energy into spiritual energy

Dukha Sanskrit term, which translated means suffering or pain. Yogi and Buddhist philosophy describes all life as suffering or pain
Dharana One of the eight limbs of yoga, focusing on meditation practice. Concentration – the sixth limb of yoga
Dharma Righteous conduct
Dhyana One of the eight limbs of yoga, focusing on meditation practice. Meditation – the seventh limb of yoga
Dvesa One of the klesas. Hatred or dislike

Ego The false aspect of ourselves and our persona, the mask, the seeker of pleasure and avoider of pain
Exercise The term exercise describes physical activity that is planned, structured and performed regularly to achieve a specific goal, for example: to improve fitness and/or health; to assist the management of a medical condition; to feel better; to lose weight. Exercise may involve going to the gym, going for a run, walk, cycle or a swim, or attending a group exercise or yoga session

Granthi Knot. Protective mechanisms in the sushumna to prevent upward flowing of prana and protect the individual from an energy overload

Guna Quality of nature and the universe. Quality of mind

Guru Teacher

Gurukula System by which the student lives with their guru or teacher

Hatha yoga Physical yoga and the practice of asanas or postures/positions to improve strength and flexibility. The aim being to unite the right and left energies and merge with sushumna

Hatha Yoga Pradipika One of the main scriptures that explains Hatha yoga practice. Compiled in the fifteenth century by the sage Svatmarama

High density lipo-protein – HDL Healthy cholesterol

Iyengar yoga One approach to Hatha yoga, developed by B.K.S. Iyengar, one of the most influential teachers of yoga in the western world

Ida Left side nadi: feminine, intuitive, holistic, cool, subjective. Terminates at the left nostril

Jalandhara bandha Throat or chin lock, which forces prana downwards

Japa Repetition of a mantra

Jnana Knowledge

Kapalabhati Kriya, a cleansing breathing exercise, means shining skull

Karma The law of cause and effect

Karma yoga Spiritual yoga pathway; selfless service to God

Klesha Blocks, sorrows or afflictions to be overcome through yoga. Caused by egoism, desire, ignorance and hatred

Kriya Action. Cleansing or purifying technique

Kriya yoga Yoga of purifying action, as taught by Patanjali

Khumbaka Retention of breath

Kundalini Primordial, divine cosmic energy located in all individuals

Laya Absorption of the mind

Liberation The aim of all forms and approaches to 'yoga' practice. Freeing the self from the illusions of the mind and ego and experiencing the connection of head, heart and spirit

Low Density lipo-protein – LDL Unhealthy cholesterol

Mahatma Sacred and great soul

Maha-Samadhi Leaving the body for the final time to become one with God

Manipuraka chakra Solar plexus chakra site, which locates fear and apprehension

Manomaya kosha One of the five sheaths or layers of the astral body. The psychological sheath

Mantra Sacred symbol or syllable, word or words. Used for chanting

Mudra Seals, using the hands

Muladhara chakra Root chakra. Controls sexual energy

Moola Anal lock forcing the energy upwards

Nadis Energy channels through which prana moves

Niyama One of the eight limbs of yoga, focusing on ethical and spiritual yoga practices (see also, Yama). Personal observance and discipline, with the aim to develop five aspects:
- Purity
- Contentment
- Discipline
- Study
- Devotion

OM Pranava or sacred symbol (monosyllable) representing Atman and Brahman. A chant used at the beginning and end of prayers. OM. God, I am. At one with the divine

Patanjali Author who compiled the Yoga Sutras, one of the six Indian schools of philosophy and which informs Buddhist philosophy

Physical activity The term physical activity describes all human movement that increases energy expenditure above resting level. This includes:
- Everyday activities: DIY, housework, gardening, active travel (walking or cycling), active play and recreational activities
- Active leisure and recreation: exercise classes, gym sessions, swimming, dance, yoga, pilates etc.
- Sport: games and athletics; either recreational or competitive (DoH, 2011)

Pingala Right side nadi: masculine, logical, aggressive, hot. Terminates at the right nostril

Prana The 'life energy' that travels around the body through channels (nadis). The life force in all things

Pranava The scared symbol, Om

Pranayama One of the eight limbs of yoga, focusing on breath and control, and breathing exercises, as practised in Hatha yoga. Their aim is to release energy blockages and activate Kundalini energy

Pranamaya kosha One of the five sheaths or layers of the astral body

Pratyahara One of the eight limbs of yoga, focusing on meditation practice. Fifth limb. Withdrawing the senses

Raja Yoga Royal yoga, silencing the thoughts and realising the true nature. Raja yoga focuses on harnessing the mind

through meditation practice. The goal is unity with the higher power. Raja yoga contains Patajali's eight limbs
Rajas Guna, energy, stimulation, restlessness
Raga One of the kleshas. Attachment or desire
Rig veda Oldest of the vedas
Rigpa A state free of full relaxation, free of all mental constructions
Rishi Seer

Sahasara chakra Crown chakra. Thousand lotus petals, located at the crown of the head. The most important chakra; once uncoiled the seeker is brought to freedom
Santosha One of the Niyamas – meaning contentment
Samskara Habitual movement of the mind
Samadhi One of the eight limbs of yoga, focusing on meditation practice. Absorption and self-realisation. The eighth limb, the super conscious state
Sankaracharaya Ninth-century philosopher and leading exponent of Advaita (non-dualism) Vedanta; founder of the Swami order of monks
Satsang Spiritual meeting
Sattva Purity
Sattvic Natural and organic and vegetarian food
Satya One of the yamas – meaning truthfulness
Saucha Niyama – meaning purity or cleanliness
Shanti Peace
Shakti Female goddess, the power, energy of the female
Sutra Sanskrit term, which translated means 'thread'
Sushumna Central nadi running though the centre of the spine
Svadhyaya Self-enquiry. Any study that helps an individual to understand their self. One of niyamas and part of kriya yoga
Swadhisthanana chakra Base chakra. Located behind the genitals. Site of wordly desires
Swami Hindu monk
Swamiji Affectionate term for swami

Tantra Technique
Tantra Yoga Esoteric practice of yoga. Focus on removing blocks to enable free flow of prana in sushumna
Tamas One of the gunas. Darkness, poison, laziness. Responsible for heaviness, stability

Tapas One of the niyamas – meaning austerity, penance. A component of kriya yoga. Process of removing impurities
Turiya A state where the yogi sees god everywhere

Udana One of the five major pranas, governs the throat region
Uddiyana bandha Abdominal contraction bandha
Ujjayi Advanced pranayama
Upanishads Philosophical texts written in India

Vedanta The most influential school of Indian philosophy, taught by the Swamis, including: Shivananda, Satchidananda, Vishnu Devananda
Vedas Ancient Hindu scriptures containing the Upanishads. The foundations for all yoga
Viniyoga One approach to Hatha yoga, developed by Desikachar
Vishuddha chakra Throat chakra located in the throat region. Seat of intellectual awareness
Vijnamaya kosha One of the five sheaths or layers of the astral body – the intellectual sheath
Vivekananda One of the first swamis to travel to the West
Vyana One of the five pranas. Governs the muscles, limbs and posture

Yama One of the eight limbs of yoga focusing on ethical and spiritual yoga practices (see also, Niyama). Ethics and ways to live. Dealings with society and the world. Self restraint which includes restraint from five aspects:
- Non-violence
- Non-lying
- Not stealing
- Sexual moderation
- Not being greedy

Yoga Sanskrit term, which translated means 'unite or connect'. The path that integrates the mind, body, senses, intellect with the self
Yoga Sutra Patanjali's classical yoga text
Yogi A person who is adept at yoga, a student or a seeker of truth
Yuga Division of time. We are currently in the Kali Yuga

APPENDICES

APPENDIX 1: PASSIVE RELAXATION SCRIPT 1

- Breathe slowly and deeply
- Allow the abdominals to rise as you inhale and fall as you exhale
- Maintain a focus on softer, deeper and slower breathing
- Relax the feet, allow the feet to relax and let go, the feet are relaxed
- Relax the ankles, allow the ankles to relax and let go, the ankles are relaxed
- Relax the shins, allow the shins to relax and let go, the shins are relaxed
- Relax the knees, allow the knees to relax and let go, the knees are relaxed
- Relax the thighs, allow the thighs to relax and let go, the thighs are relaxed
- Relax the hips and buttocks, allow the hips and buttocks to relax and let go, the hips and buttocks are relaxed
- Allow the legs to surrender to the floor, the lower body is relaxed
- Relax the lower back and abdomen, allow the lower back and abdomen to relax and soften, the lower back and abdomen are relaxed
- Relax the spine, allow the spine to relax, lengthen and soften, the spine is long and relaxed
- Allow the trunk to surrender to the floor, the trunk of the body is relaxed
- Relax the shoulders, allow the shoulders to relax and soften, the shoulders are relaxed
- Relax the arms, allow the arms to soften and sink into the floor, the arms are relaxed
- Allow the shoulders and arms to surrender to the floor, the arms are relaxed
- Relax the face, allow the facial muscles to soften, relax the forehead, relax the eye sockets and eyebrows, relax the cheek bones, relax the nose, relax the mouth and the jaw, soften the tongue, the facial muscles are all soft and relaxed
- Release any tension in the scalp, relax the scalp, the scalp is relaxed
- Relax, relax, relax
- Surrender, surrender, surrender
- Relax the body
- Release all tension
- Let go
- Breathe

Allow a short period of silence and stillness and then progressively bring the body back to a more awakened state, by performing a whole body stretch and some other lying, mobilising postures. Progressively bring the body to a seated position for meditation and pranayama practice. The class can then end with meditation, pranayama or prayers/ending affirmations.

APPENDIX 2: ACTIVE RELAXATION SCRIPT

- Sit or lie in a comfortable position and allow your body to relax and lengthen
- Allow the muscles to soften
- Focus your awareness on your breathing. Notice the depth and pace of your breathing
- Allow your breath to become slower, softer and deeper

- Take your mind's awareness to your body, starting with the feet
- Spread and separate your toes, feeling the tension in the feet
- Flex your toes towards your knees, feeling the tension in the lower leg
- Stay aware of the tension, breathe steadily in and out
- Then let the toes and feet relax, let go of any tension in the lower legs
- Be still and breathe softly and deeply
- Take your mind's awareness to the thigh muscles
- Allow the muscles at the front of the thigh to tighten without locking the knee
- Tighten the muscles at the back of the thigh
- Squeeze the buttocks tight
- Stay aware of the tension in the thighs and buttocks, breathe steadily in and out
- Then let the thigh and buttock muscles relax
- Feel the hip joint open and soften
- Feel the whole of the legs relax and soften
- Be still and breathe softly and deeply
- Focus your mind's awareness to the abdomen
- Draw the abdominal muscles in tightly towards your backbone
- Feel the sides of the abdomen draw in tight
- Feel the muscles of the lower back tighten
- Stay aware of the tension, experience the feeling of a corset tightening around the centre of the body, breathe steadily in and out
- Then release the tension in these muscles, feel the centre of the body relax and let go
- Be still and breathe softly and deeply
- Focus your awareness on the shoulders and upper back
- Squeeze the shoulders towards the ears
- Feel the tension increase in the muscles of the upper back and the back of the neck, breathe steadily in and out
- Then allow the muscles to let go and release
- Lengthen the ears away from the shoulders
- Feel the chin tucking towards the body
- Feel the muscles in between the shoulder blades drawing downwards and tightening
- Stay aware of the tension, breathe steadily in and out
- Then release the tension in these muscles, allow the body to let go
- Be still and breathe softly and deeply
- Focus your awareness on the muscles of the arms
- Extend the arms and tense all the muscles in the upper and lower arms, breathe steadily in and out
- Clench the fists to increase the tension
- Stay aware of the tension, breathing steadily in and out
- Then allow the muscles to release and let go
- Spread the fingers and open up the hands
- Extend the fingers as far away from the shoulders as you can
- Stay aware of the tension in the muscles of the hands and arms, breathe steadily in and out
- Then release and let go and allow the arms to soften and relax
- Allow the body to be still, breathe slowly and deeply
- Focus your mind's awareness on the face and head
- Open your mouth wide and feel the tension around the mouth and jaw
- Stay aware of the tension, breathe steadily in and out
- Then release and let go, allow the jaw to relax, wiggle the jaw a little
- Stick out your tongue, then allow it to relax back into your mouth
- Feel the tongue soften and the mouth and jaw relax, breathe steadily in and out
- Wiggle your nose and then release
- Feel the eye sockets opening and then release

- Move the muscles in the forehead, then allow then to soften and relax
- Let the body sink deeper and relax further
- Any tension just eases away
- Tighten the whole body one last time, extending your head and toes and fingers as far away from each other as you can
- Release and let go, allow yourself to sigh
- Take your mind's awareness back to your breathing
- Focus on slower, deeper breathing
- Allow your body to be still and silent
- With every breath allow the body to relax further
- Allow a feeling of relaxation and calm to spread through your whole body.

APPENDIX 3: PASSIVE RELAXATION SCRIPT 2

- Sit or lie in a comfortable position
- Allow your body to relax and lengthen
- Allow the muscles to soften
- Focus your awareness on your breathing
- Notice the depth and pace of your breathing
- Allow your breath to become slower, softer and deeper
- Take your mind's awareness to your body, starting with the feet
- Allow the feet to soften and relax, let go of any tension
- Allow the ankle joint to open and relax
- Feel the calf muscles and muscles at the front of the shin soften
- Take a deeper breathe and on the outward breathe allow the lower leg to relax and soften even further
- Take your minds awareness to the knee joint
- Allow the knee joint to open and relax
- Feel the muscles at the front of the thigh soften
- Feel the muscles at the back of the thigh lengthen and relax
- Take a deeper breathe and on the outward breathe allow the whole of the legs to relax and let go
- Focus your mind's awareness to the hip joint
- Allow the hip joint to open up and relax
- Feel the buttock muscles relax and soften
- Feel the muscles around the hip release and open
- Focus your mind's awareness on the spine
- Start at the base of the spine and be mindful of each vertebra up to the skull
- Feel each vertebrae open up
- Allow the muscles around the vertebrae (spine) to relax and lengthen
- Allow all the tension to ease away
- Allow the shoulder blades to separate and open up
- Take a deep breath and allow the whole spine to lengthen and relax
- Focus on the abdominal muscles
- Allow them to release
- Notice how the breath fills the abdominal area
- Observe the abdomen rising and falling with each breath
- Notice the ribcage and the breastbone
- Feel the muscles around the ribs relax
- Allow the breath to become slower and deeper
- Allow the ribs and the breastbone to soften
- Focus your awareness on the shoulder joint
- Allow the shoulder joint to open up and relax
- Feel the muscles of the upper arm lengthen and relax
- Notice the elbow joint
- Feel the elbow joint relaxing and opening
- Feel the muscles of the forearm relax and soften
- Notice the wrists and the hands
- Allow the tension to ease away
- Allow the fingers to curl open and the tension

- to float away
- Focus your mind's awareness on the head
- Allow each of the facial muscles to soften and relax
- Feel the jaw relax
- Feel the tongue soften
- Feel the lips gently touching and forming a soft smile
- Allow the cheekbones to relax
- Notice the eye sockets relaxing
- Allow the forehead to relax
- Any tension just easing away
- Feel your body soften
- Allow your body to feel light and relaxed
- Take your mind's awareness back to your breathing
- Focus on slower, deeper breathing
- With every breath allow the body to relax further
- Allow a feeling of peace and calm to spread through your whole body.

APPENDIX 4: HEALING RELAXATION SCRIPT

- Sit or lie in a comfortable position
- Allow your body to relax and be still
- Allow the muscles to soften and lengthen
- Notice any sensations that arise anywhere in the body
- Acknowledge these, ask what they need, pay attention
- Avoid any judgement, just stay aware and sensitive to the messages the body sends
- Bring the focus of your awareness to your breathing
- Notice the depth and pace of your breathing
- Allow your breath to become slower, softer and deeper
- Inhale through the nose, exhale through the nose
- Allow the abdominal area to rise as you inhale and fall as you exhale
- Inhale and feel the breath travelling down to the abdomen
- Exhale and feel the breath flowing upwards and out of the body
- Stay connected to the sensations and feelings in the body
- Give permission for the body to relax and let go
- Breathe in love
- Breathe out tension
- Breathe in harmony
- Breathe out discord
- Breathe in healing
- Breathe out disease
- Stay focused on the breath
- Allow the breath to become slower and deeper
- Breathe in love
- Breathe out tension
- Breathe in harmony
- Breathe out discord
- Breathe in healing
- Breathe out disease
- Release all self judgement and criticism
- Focus on breathing in joy and love
- Focus on allowing the body to heal
- Allow the thoughts to assist healing
- Release and let go of any blocks to well-being, allow yourself to sigh, let go
- Focus on slower, deeper breathing
- Release all self-judgement and criticism
- Breathe in love
- Breathe out tension
- Breathe in harmony
- Breathe out discord
- Breathe in healing
- Breathe out disease
- Allow your body to be still and silent
- Allow the body to share what it needs to heal

- With every breath allow the body to relax further
- Allow a feeling of relaxation and calm to spread through your whole body
- Be here and now
- Allow the body and mind to flow together creating a sense of peace and well-being.

APPENDIX 5: SIMPLE CHAKRA MEDITATION

- Sit in a comfortable position, e.g. Sukhasana, cross-legged pose
- Allow your body to relax and be still
- Allow the muscles to soften and lengthen
- Allow the breath to deepen and become slower
- As you inhale abdominals rise, as you exhale abdominals fall

- Focus on the root chakra – muladhara, located at the perineum at the bottom of the spine
- Visualise the chakra as a circle of red light, spiralling and connecting down into the earth
- Repeat the mantra Lam

- Focus on the base or sacral chakra – svadshistana, located in the pelvis, just below the navel
- Visualise the chakra as an orange circle of light, spiralling forwards from the body
- Repeat the mantra Vam

- Focus on the solar plexus chakra – manipura, located in the navel, the power chakra
- Visualise the chakra as a yellow circle of light spiralling forwards from the navel
- Repeat the mantra Ram

- Focus on the heart chakra – anahata, located at the heart centre
- Visualise the chakra as a green or pink light, spiralling forwards from the heart
- Repeat the mantra Yam

- Focus on the throat chakra – Visuddha, located in the throat region, the communication chakra, I speak my truth
- Visualise the chakra as a turquoise light, spiralling forwards from the throat
- Repeat the mantra Ham

- Focus on the third eye chakra – ajna, between the eyebrows, the intuition chakra
- Visualise the chakra as a purple light, spiralling forwards from the forehead
- Repeat the mantra Ksham

- Focus on the crown chakra – sahasara, slightly above the top of the head
- Visualise the chakra as a golden or white light, spiralling upwards towards the heavens
- Repeat the mantra Om

- Feel the connection of all chakras
- Chant the mantras – Lam, Vam, Ram, Yam, Ham, Ksham, Om (repeat chant for desired number of cycles)
- Focus on the breath and stillness.

Final word

Just as a person casts off worn out clothes and puts on new ones, so also the embodied self casts off worn out bodies and enters others which are new. (Bhagavad Gita 2.22)

From: Swami Saradananda (2010)

INDEX

Abhinivesha 45
activity guidelines 195
adapt, adjust and accommodate 212–13
Ahimsa 19–20, 215
apana 31, 32
Aparigraha 21
asanas 18, 23, 57–147, 201
    aims/benefits of 57–8
    backward-bending postures 105–16
    definition of 57
    forward-bending postures 95–104
    inverted postures 140–7
    laterally extending postures 85–9
    practice of 58–61
    seated asanas 117–31
    standing/balancing postures 61–77
    strengthening postures 90–5
    supine lying asanas 132–9
    twisting postures 78–84
    POSES AND BANDHAS
    abdominal lock (Uddiyana Bandha) 166, 167
    adept pose/perfect pose (Siddhasana) 118–19
    belly twist (Jathara Parivartanasana) 137
    boat pose (Navasana) 123
    bow pose (Dhanurasana) 105–6
    bridge pose (Setu Bandhasana) 110–11
    camel pose (Ustrasana) 112–13
    chair pose/fierce pose (Utkatasana) 73
    child's pose (Balasana) 139
    cobbler's pose (Baddhakonasana) 124
    cobra pose (Bhujangasana) 106–7
    corpse pose (Savasana) 134
    cow face posture (Gomukasana) 131
    crane pose/crow pose (Bakasana) 145
    dancer's pose/King of the dance pose (Natarajasana) 76–7
    downward-facing dog (Adho Mukha Shvanasana) 140–1
    downward-facing hero pose (Adho Mukha Virasana) 127
    eagle pose (Garudasana) 74
    easy pose/cross-legged pose (Sukhasana) 117
    extended hand to big toe pose (Uttihita Hasta Padangusthasana) 75–6

extended side stretch (Utthita Parsvakonasana) 85–6
fish pose (Matsyasana) 116
four-limbed staff pose/crocodile pose (Chaturanga Dandasana) 92
great lock (Maha Bandha) 169
half lord of the fishes pose (Ardha Matsyendrasana) 84
half lotus pose (Ardha Padmasana) 120
half moon pose (Ardha Chandrasana) 86–7
half shoulder stand (Ardha Sarvangasana) 142
half wind-relieving pose (Ardha Apanasana) 136
head stand (Sirsasana) 146–7
head to knee pose (Janu Sirsasana) 102–3
hero pose (Virasana/Vajrasana) 125
legs up the wall pose (Viparita Karani) 133
lion pose (Simhasana) 130
locust pose (Shalabasana) 109
lotus pose (Padmasana) 121
marichi's pose/sage's pose (Marichyasana) 129
garland pose/Hindi squat pose/frog pose (Malasana) 72
mountain pose (Tadasana) 62–3
plank (Khumbhakasana) 91
plough (Halasana) 144
reclined cobbler's pose (Supta Baddhakonasana) 138
reclined hero pose (Supta Virasana) 128
revolved head to knee pose (Parivrtta Janu Sirsasana) 88–9
revolved triangle pose (Parivrtta Trikonasana) 82–3
root lock/perineum or cervix lock (Moola Bandha) 166, 168
same angle posture/right angle posture (Samokonasana) 100
side plank pose/T stand (Vasishthasana) 93–4
side twist in the hero pose (Parsva Virasana) 126
single leg forward bend (Parsvottanasana) 101–2
shoulder stand (Sarvangasana) 143
staff pose (Dandasana) 122
standing forward bend (Uttanasana) 96–7
throat or chin lock (Jalandhara Bandha) 166
tree pose (Vrkshasana) 65–6
triangle pose (Uttihita Trikonasana) 80–1
twisting chair pose (Parivrtta Utkutasana) 79

upward-facing dog pose (Urdhva Mukha Shvanasana) 108
upward-facing plank/intense east side stretch (Purvottanasana) 94–5
upward salute/raised hand pose (Urdhva Hastasana) 64
warrior poses (Virabhadrasanas) 66–71
wheel pose/upward-facing bow (Chakrasana) 114–15
wide-angle seated forward bend (Upavistha Konasana) 104
wide-legged forward bend (Prasarita Padottanasana) 98–9
wind-relieving pose/knees to chest pose (Apanasana) 135
ashramas 26
ashtanga vinyasa krama yoga 55–6
ashtanga vinyasa yoga 59–60
ashtanga yoga 19–24, 212, 216
asmita 45
asteya 20
asthma 208–9
avidya 9, 12, 36, 37, 42, 44, 45
Ayurveda 41, 163

back pain, non-specific lower (LBP) 205–6
bandhas 165–9
Bhagavad Gita 10, 11, 21, 24–6
bhakti yoga 11, 17, 25, 214–16
Bihar school of yoga 56
bikram yoga 56
body warming 174
brahmacharya 20–1
breath control, *see* pranayama
breathing techniques 149–51, 166
    alternate nostril breathing (anuloma viloma) 161
    alternate nostril breathing (nadi sodhana) 155
    bellows breathing (bhastrika) 160
    cooling breath (sithali) 157
    cooling or hissing breath (sitkari) 158
    deep abdominal breathing (corpse pose) 152
    full yogic breath 153
    hummingbee (brahmari breath) 154
    lung-cleansing exercise (kapalabhati) 156
    vitality stimulating breath (surya bhedana) 159

cardiovascular fitness 196, 199
caste system 14
chakras 32, 33, 34–6, 38–9, 163, 236
chanting, *see* mantras
chronic obstructive pulmonary disease (COPD) 208
counterposes (pratikriyasana) 59, 188–9

depression 202
devotion 212
dharana 23, 46
dhyana 23–4, 46
diabetes 207
doshas 40, 41, 170–1
drishti 59–60
dvesha 45

ego (ahamkara) 42, 212–13, 215
emotional fitness 195

flexibility 196–7, 199

Gayatri mantra remembering sequence 50
general anxiety disorder (GAD) 202
granthis 36–7
gratitude 215–16
gunas 26

Hatha yoga 12, 17–18, 53–6
    breathing 60–1
    counterposes (pratikriyasana) 59, 188–9
    full/main poses 59
    lineages 55–6
    preparation poses 58–9
    see also Hatha yoga session structure
Hatha Yoga Pradipika (HYP) 18, 37, 53
    asanas 57, 118, 119
    bandhas 166, 168, 169
    mudras 162, 165
    pranayama 148, 149, 154
Hatha yoga session structure 58–9, 172–91
    preparatory phase 172–85
    main phase 186–9
    closing phase 189–91
health and total fitness model 194–6
householder path 20–1, 26, 198–9, 212
hypertension 209–10

ida 34, 35, 36, 53
intelligence (buddhi) 42
ishwara pranidhana 12, 22–3, 46
Iyengar yoga 55

jala neti (nasal cleansing) 170
jihva dhauti (tongue scraping) 171
jnana yoga 11, 25, 164, 216–17

kapalabhati (shining skull) 156, 171
karma yoga 10–11, 25, 215
kleshas 45–6
koshas 28–34
kriya yoga 12, 45–6
kriyas 170–1
kumbaka breathing/breath retention 150–1, 166
kundalini 35, 36, 37, 53
kundalini yoga 12, 162–3

mantras 11, 49–52, 214, 217, 236
medical fitness 195
meditation 43, 44, 46–9, 51–2, 117, 190, 201, 236
mental fitness 195
mental health 200–1
mind (manas) 41–5, 212
mindfulness 43, 201, 217–18
mobility/mobilisation (pawanmuktasana) 173–4
moksha (liberation) 16, 26, 150
motor fitness 197–8, 199
mudras 162–5
muscular fitness 197, 199

nadis 34, 35
namaste 164–5
nauli (abdominal churning/massage) 171
niyamas 22–3
nutrition 200
nutritional fitness 194–5

obesity/overweight 206
Om 51–2
osteoarthritis 203–4
osteoporosis 202–3

palmistry 163
panch maya koshas 28–34
Patanjali 13, 42, 46
    yoga sutras 16, 18–19, 20, 23, 24, 57, 213
perception 44–5
physical fitness 194, 196–8, 199
physical health 200
pingala 34, 35, 36, 53
positive outlook 213–14
prana, and energetic body 28–34
pranava mantra 51–2
pranayama 23, 60–1, 148–61, 190–1, 201: *see also* breathing techniques

pratyahara 23, 46

raga 45
raja yoga 11, 18, 25
relaxation 18, 173, 189–90
relaxation scripts 232–6
rheumatoid arthritis 204–5

samadhi 24, 46, 53
samana 31, 32
samavrtti (same action breathing) 149–50
samyama 24, 212
santosha 22, 212
satya 20
satyananda yoga 56
saucha 22
self-realisation 36
senses 42, 211–12
service 215, 217
shad darsanas 13
sharira 27–8
sivananda yoga 55
social fitness 195–6
spiritual fitness 196
spiritual health 201
sushumna 34, 35, 36, 53
svadhyaha 12, 22, 46

tantra yoga 12, 16
tapas 12, 22, 46
trataka/tratakam (concentrated gazing) 171
turiya 51–2

udana 31, 32
ujjayi breathing/victorious breath 150
Upanishads 15–16

Vedas 14–15, 184
viniyoga 55
vinyasa yoga 55, 187–8
vyana 32, 34

yamas 19–21
yoga
    and chronic health conditions 200–10
    definition of 9, 13
    8 limbs of 19–24
    history of 13–18

    and lifestyle 198–200
    paths of 9–10
    philosophy of 7–8, 13, 211–18
yoga sequences 219–26
    cat pose (Marjaryasana) to cow pose (bitilasana) 179–80
    focus sequence 224
    forward bend and sukhasana purvottasana 178
    hip opening sequence 221
    preparation for meditation sequence 225
    salute to Lord Shiva 222
    seated mobilisation 177
    seated mobilisation with affection sequence 226
    shankaprakshalana (digestive cleansing sequence) 219–20
    standing easy sequence (warming) 185
    strength sequence 223
    sun salutations (surya namsakara) 180–4
    supine mobilisation 175–6
yoga sutras 16, 18–19, 20, 23, 24, 44, 57, 148, 149, 213
yoga therapy 18
yogic diet 200